COMPLETE
BOOK OF FORMS
FOR THE
SCHOOL HEALTH
PROFESSIONAL

JERRY NEWTON, M.D.

Director, School Health Services
San Antonio Independent School District
San Antonio, Texas

PRENTICE HALL
Englewood Cliffs, New Jersey 07632

Prentice-Hall International, Inc., *London*
Prentice-Hall of Australia, Pty. Ltd., *Sydney*
Prentice-Hall Canada, Inc., *Toronto*
Prentice-Hall of India Private Ltd., *New Delhi*
Prentice-Hall of Japan, Inc., *Tokyo*
Prentice-Hall of Southeast Asia Pte. Ltd., *Singapore*
Editora Prentice-Hall do Brasil Ltda., *Rio de Janeiro*
Prentice-Hall Hispanoamericana, S.A., *Mexico*

Library of Congress Cataloging-in-Publication Data

Newton, Jerry,
  Complete book of forms for the school health
professional.

  Includes index.
  1. School hygiene—United States—Forms.
2. School nursing—United States—Forms.   I. Title.
[DNLM: 1. School Health Services—United States—
forms. WA 350 N5715c]
LB3405.N45   1987   371.7   87-13944

ISBN 0-13-156498-6

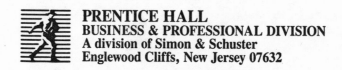

PRENTICE HALL
BUSINESS & PROFESSIONAL DIVISION
A division of Simon & Schuster
Englewood Cliffs, New Jersey 07632

Printed in the United States of America.

ABOUT THE AUTHOR

Jerry Newton, a pediatrician with a wide variety of experiences, conducted a busy private practice in San Antonio, Texas, for 23 years. This was followed by 3 years of bouncing around in a jeep as a Peace Corps physician in Paraguay, where he not only was the personal physician to 75 Peace Corps volunteers, but also the medical supervisor for the Peace Corps Public Health Program in Paraguay.

On returning to the United States, Dr. Newton became the full-time medical director of the San Antonio Independent School District and has been serving in that position for over 12 years. Many school districts have medical consultants but in only a few is the physician an active member of the superintendent's staff. Moving through the corridors of 90 schools, and constant contact with school nurses, principals, and teachers, have given him an unusual insight into the special medical problems of school children and the need for better health education.

He has consistently applied his efforts to improve the quality of health care offered to students. To increase the effectiveness and expand the services provided by school nurses, he developed an active school nurse practitioner program, which has resulted in many newer and innovative school health programs and clinics dealing with learning disabilities and behavior problems.

Dr. Newton is clinical professor of pediatrics at the University of Texas Medical School in San Antonio and has been active in school health committees of his local and state medical associations as well as the American School Health Association and the American Academy of Pediatrics. He is also the author of *School Health Handbook: A Ready Reference for School Nurses and Educators* (Prentice-Hall, 1984).

ABOUT THIS BOOK

Complete Book of Forms for the School Health Professional is for all school health personnel who spend a large part of their time on paperwork, which reduces the time available for health services or health education. Under the best of systems, school health forms will always be required—some mandated by the state, others by the local school district. Large school districts use more forms and often develop numbered, coded, and indexed forms for their own use. In smaller districts, each school principal or school nurse may develop a few forms as needed. Many smaller districts, however, do not have access to medical or nursing consultation and, thus, lack the expertise required to assure that the school health-related forms not only provide for the health needs of the students, but also meet state reporting requirements.

This book has been compiled to help all school districts develop appropriate school health forms or to modify their existing forms when necessary. Included are examples of over 245 school health forms that are used throughout the United States. While it is unlikely that all these forms would be suitable for any one district, all districts could use some of them, usually in a format adapted to their particular needs.

Some forms may suggest new health programs that have not been used by your district but are beneficial for the children and simple to carry out. Examples of these forms are scoliosis screening and the expansion of vision screening to include testing for eye muscle imbalance.

In a source book of this nature, the ease of finding the desired form is of prime importance. For your convenience, the forms have been arranged according to subject matter. Forms used for physical referral, annual reports, parental release/permission/notification, screening procedures, health appraisals, and so on will be found under the appropriate subject matter heading, including Immunization, Medications, Vision, Hearing, and Child Abuse. To help you see how certain forms are completed, a filled-in sample follows several of the blank forms. Several of the forms are also given in Spanish.

Included are variations of forms that are frequently used, ranging from all-inclusive long forms to specific and brief ones. This affords each school district the opportunity to select and make as many copies as necessary of the forms shown or develop a composite that best suits local needs.

Intended for professionally trained health personnel, some of the forms may be confusing to health aides or licensed vocational (or practical) nurses. Since some smaller districts rely solely on these paraprofessionals to carry out the health program, the more complicated forms are explained in detail so that nonprofessional personnel may understand and use them.

Thus, *Complete Book of Forms for the School Health Professional* should help increase the understanding and dialogue among school health professionals, teachers, physicians, and parents so that each child's health and well-being can be served.

Jerry Newton, M.D.

ACKNOWLEDGMENTS

The forms in this book are either adaptations or copies of those used in many school districts across the United States. Some are from my own district, and some I designed for this book.

I am grateful to the many school nurse coordinators who shared their districts' forms with me. I also wish to thank the medical societies, athletic departments, state health departments, individual researchers, printing companies, and pharmaceutical houses who gave me permission to use forms they have developed and/or printed. The following is a list of all these sources:

ABC Unified School District, Cerritos, CA (Betty McGinnis, RN)

Arizona Department Health Services, Tempe, AZ (Bette Denlinger, RN)

Arizona Interscholastic Association, Phoenix, AZ

Bassett Unified School District, La Puente, CA (Baalah Drooks, RN)

Dallas Independent School District, Dallas, TX (Marilyn Marcontel, RN)

K/P Graphics, Roseland, CA

Los Angeles County Office of Education, Downey, CA (Susan Lordi, RN)

Minneapolis State High School League, Anoka, MN

Montebello Unified School District, Montebello, CA (G. A. Ristic, RN)

New Hampshire Department of Education, Concord, NH (Muriel Desrosiers, RN)

New Hampshire Medical Society, Concord, NH

Oklahoma Secondary School Activities Association, Oklahoma City, OK

Palos Verdes ISD, Palos Verdes, CA (Marjorie Harrison, RN)

Pomona Unified School District, Pomona, CA (Beth Hadady, RN)

Rena Ullman and co-workers for the ACTeRS Chart

Ross Laboratories for the height/weight charts and grids

San Antonio Independent School District, San Antonio, TX

Texas Education Agency, Austin, TX (Sunny Thomas, RN)

I also wish to thank the editorial staff at Prentice-Hall, Evelyn Fazio and Diane Turso, who helped with suggestions and technical assistance.

Finally, I am happy to acknowledge the large part Rose, my wife and chief critic, played in designing, typing, and putting together the various loose ends that have to be coordinated in this kind of book.

CONTENTS

section three
FORMS FOR ATHLETICS AND
PHYSICAL EDUCATION   21

section four
FORMS FOR CHILD ABUSE   35

section five
FORMS FOR COMMUNICABLE DISEASE   41

section six
FORMS FOR THE DENTAL PROGRAM   55

section seven
FORMS FOR EVALUATION
AND OBSERVATION OF
SCHOOL NURSES AND AIDES   59

section eight
FORMS FOR HEALTH FILE
FOR EACH STUDENT

section nine
FORMS FOR HISTORY OF HEALTH
AND DEVELOPMENT

section ten
FORMS FOR HEARING SCREENINGS AND TESTING 105

section eleven
FORMS FOR HEIGHT AND WEIGHT 119

section twelve
FORMS FOR IMMUNIZATIONS

129

section thirteen
FORMS FOR MEDICATION

151

section fourteen
FORMS FOR NURSE'S REPORTS

167

section fifteen
FORMS FOR PARENT INFORMATION, NOTIFICATION, AND RELEASE OF INFORMATION

191

section sixteen
FORMS FOR PHYSICAL EXAMINATIONS AND NURSE ASSESSMENTS 207

section seventeen
FORMS FOR PREGNANT STUDENTS   **233**

section eighteen
FORMS FOR SCOLIOSIS   **239**

section nineteen
FORMS FOR SPECIAL EDUCATION LIAISON   **253**

section twenty
FORMS FOR SPECIAL
NURSING PROCEDURES

301

section twenty-one
FORMS FOR SUPPLIES   313

section twenty-two
FORMS FOR TEACHER-NURSE
CONSULTATIONS   319

section twenty-three
FORMS FOR VISION   **329**

FORMS FOR
ACCIDENTS
AND EMERGENCIES

All school districts have (or should have) official policy procedures governing how accidents and emergencies at school should be handled, documented, and reported.

Here is an example of one school district's procedures:

I. All accidents involving pupils on the school grounds or in the building shall be reported to the principal. If prompt treatment is believed necessary, the parent or guardian shall be called and shall assume responsibility for further decisions.

If, in the judgment of the principal and/or the school nurse, the pupil is in immediate danger and the parent or guardian cannot be located to assume responsibility and if there is no official parental authorization, the principal or the school nurse shall have the pupil taken to the emergency room of the Medical Center Hospital, unless the principal or the nurse knows that the pupil will be accepted at a hospital that is less distant. The principal and/or the nurse shall decide whether the child should be transported by private automobile or whether the local emergency ambulance service should be called. The person taking the pupil to the hospital shall remain with the pupil until the parent or guardian arrives. If a private car is used, two adults should be assigned, allowing one person to attend the student.

II. Guidelines for rendering first aid
First aid is to be administered in accordance with procedures outlined in the
A. *American Red Cross Handbook.*
B. *The County Medical Society's Handbook for School Health Aides.*

C. Department of School Health Services, *Handbook of Administrative Procedures and Programs,* Section on Medical Protocols.

III. Consent to medical treatment

The principal or designate is, by law, authorized to consent to emergency medical treatment for a student provided that prior written authorization has been obtained from the parent or legal guardian.

A. The school in which a minor student is enrolled shall consent to medical treatment of the student provided that

1. The person having the power to consent as otherwise provided by law cannot be contacted.
2. Actual notice to the contrary has not been given by that person.
3. Written authorization to consent has been received from that person.

B. Consent to medical treatment under this policy shall be in writing, signed by the school official giving consent, and given to the doctor, hospital, or other medical facility that administers the treatment. The consent must contain

1. The name of the student.
2. The name of one or both parents, if known, and the name of the managing conservator or guardian of the student, if either has been appointed.
3. The name of the school official giving consent and his or her relation to the student.
4. A statement of the nature of the medical treatment to be given.
5. The date on which the treatment is to begin.

IV. Reporting requirements

A. Completion of accident report

1. This form is to be used in cases of injuries that are serious enough to require more than first aid attention.
2. It shall be the principal's responsibility to decide whether or not to file an accident report. School professionals, such as a campus nurse, teacher, counselor, coach, and so on, may complete *all* sections of the form.
3. The accident report may be filled out by the professional school nurse. If the school does not have a campus nurse that day, the Central Health Office should be called to send one as soon as possible.
4. A health aide may fill out the student identifying information section on the form, but it must be reviewed and signed by a school professional.

B. Distribution of the accident report form

The form is to be completed by the close of the school day and distributed, one copy to each of the following:

1. Parents
2. Department of School Health Services
3. School principal

Many of the daily accidents at school are serious enough to be recorded and reported. Reports should be brief and objective.

It is usually simpler for someone without a medical background to use a check-off sheet, as shown in the second sample form. However, no matter what kind of accident report is used, all information should be accurate and precise. Here are two examples:

Example 1. Abrasion (brush burn)

Johnny fell on his knee on the sidewalk. He walked into the clinic with a slight limp. There is a round, shallow abrasion, ½″ in diameter on his left knee.

The abrasion was washed with warm water and soap. Bleeding stopped with gentle pressure, and a 4" × 4" gauze flat was applied. Parents were notified.

Example 2. Laceration (cut)

Mary fell on the gravel playground and cut her right forearm. Cut is $\frac{1}{2}$" long × $\frac{1}{8}$" wide, and about $\frac{1}{4}$" deep, just below elbow.

Washed with soap and water, applied butterfly dressing to pull edges together, covered with adhesive bandage, and notified parents.

STUDENT EMERGENCY CARD

The Student Emergency Card should be on file for *every* student and updated annually. It allows the school to act *in loco parentis* and gives legal permission to a physician to render treatment in case of emergency trauma or illness when the parent cannot be located.

Physicians will treat truly life-threatening emergencies even if this presigned consent form is not available. However, if the condition is painful but not life threatening, such as a fractured forearm, many emergency facilities will, for fear of a lawsuit, delay treatment until parents can be located.

ACCIDENT REPORT

Instructions: This form is to be used in case of injuries that are serious enough to require more than first aid attention. On the day of the accident send one copy to the parents, one copy to the central office involved, and retain one for your records.

Date _____

School _____

Name of injured _____

Address _____

Telephone number or nearest phone _____

Nature of injury _____

_____

_____

_____

What was done to render first aid? _____

_____

_____

_____

Factors involved in accident _____

_____

_____

_____

Remarks _____

_____

_____

_____

_____

Principal _____
☐ **Nurse**
☐ **Teacher** _____
☐ **Other**

ACCIDENT REPORT

_____
Name of school

INSTRUCTIONS: READ CAREFULLY. Fill in completely. Use this form to report all accidents to students that occur while they are under the jurisdiction of the school. School jurisdiction accidents unless otherwise defined by administrative or court ruling are those occurring while students are on school property, in school buildings, and on the way to and from school. The report should be made out in triplicate.

Important: It is essential that the accident be described in sufficient detail to show safe and unsafe acts and conditions existing when the accident occurred. (When possible use a checkmark.)

1. Name_____ Home address_____
2. Sex: M ☐ F ☐ Age_____ School_____ Teacher_____
3. Time of accident: Hour _____ A.M. ☐ P.M. ☐ Date _____
4. Place of accident: School building ☐ School grounds ☐ To or from school ☐ Interscholastic athletics ☐

5.

Apparent Nature of Injury

☐ Abrasion   ☐ Fracture
☐ Amputation   ☐ Laceration
☐ Bruise   ☐ Puncture
☐ Burn   ☐ Scratches
☐ Cut   ☐ Sprain
Other (specify) _____

Description of Accident and Treatment Given

How did the accident happen? What was the student doing? Where was student? List specifically unsafe acts and unsafe conditions existing. Specify any tool, machine, or equipment involved.

_____
_____
_____
_____
_____
_____

Part of Body Injured

☐ Ankle   ☐ Hand
☐ Arm   ☐ Head
☐ Back   ☐ Knee
☐ Elbow   ☐ Leg
☐ Eye   ☐ Nose
☐ Face   ☐ Scalp
☐ Finger   ☐ Tooth
☐ Foot   ☐ Wrist
Other (specify) _____

Witness's Name	Address
_____	_____
_____	_____
_____	_____

6.

Immediate Action Taken

First aid treatment   ☐ By (name) _____
Sent to school nurse   ☐ By (name) _____
Sent home   ☐ By (name) _____
Sent to physician   ☐ By (name) _____
               Physician's name _____
Sent to hospital   ☐ By (name) _____
               Name of hospital _____
               How was student transported? _____

---

7. Was the parent or other individual notified? No ☐ Yes ☐ When_____ How?_____

Name of individual notified: _____

By whom? (enter name) _____

8.

Location

Specific Activity

☐ Athletic   ☐ Dressing room   ☐ School grounds
☐ Auditorium   ☐ Gymnasium   ☐ Shop _____
☐ Classroom   ☐ Home Economics   ☐ Showers
☐ Corridor   ☐ Laboratories   ☐ Stairs
☐ Cafeteria   ☐ Other _____

_____
_____
_____

Follow-up

_____
_____
_____
_____
_____
_____

Total number of days lost from school_____
(To be completed when student returns to school.)

Date _____

Principal _____

District health assistant_____

District nurse_____

ACCIDENT REPORT

Instructions: Fill in at the time of the accident by the person caring for an injured student who is referred to a doctor.

Student name _____ Phone _____

Address _____ Age _____ Sex _____

Date _____ Time _____ Insurance _____

Grade _____ Teacher _____ School _____

Location of accident _____

Person in attendance _____

Nature of accident		Part of body injured		
Abrasion	Head injury	Abdomen	Eye*	Head
Bruise/bump	Fracture	Ankle*	Face	Knee*
Burn	Laceration	Arm*	Finger*	Leg*
Cut	Puncture	Back	Foot*	Teeth
Convulsion	Shock	Chest	Hand	Wrist*
Dislocation	Sprain	Elbow*		
Other _____		Other _____		
_____		_____		
		*Left, right, both.		

How did it happen? _____

_____

_____

_____

Were parents notified? Yes _____ No _____

Treatment and disposition _____

_____

Follow-up _____

Amount of time lost from school _____

(Signature) _____

Principal, teacher, or nurse

ANIMAL BITE REPORT

Date of bite _____ Time of bite _____

Name of person involved _____

   Address _____

   City, state, zip _____

   Telephone _____ Age _____ Sex _____

Breed/type of animal with general description _____

_____

   Age of animal _____ Sex of animal _____

   Approximate weight of animal _____

   Date of vaccination _____ City _____

Description of incident (on school grounds? to/from school? animal confined, leashed/unleashed? etc.)

_____

_____

Area on person bitten _____

Owner of animal _____

   Address _____

   City, state, zip _____

   Telephone _____

Bite reported to ___ (local animal control agency) _____

Time and date reported _____

Signature _____

HEAD INJURY SHEET

Instructions: This form should be accompanied by a telephone call or a home visit.

Dear Parent:

Today, _____ received an injury to the head. Your child was seen in the clinic and had no problems at that time, but you should watch for any of the following symptoms:

1. Severe headache.

2. Excessive drowsiness (awake the child at least twice during the night).

3. Nausea and/or vomiting.

4. Double vision, blurred vision, or pupils of different sizes.

5. Loss of muscle coordination such as falling down, walking strangely, or staggering.

6. Any unusual behavior such as being confused, breathing irregularly, or being dizzy.

7. Convulsion.

8. Bleeding or discharge from an ear, nose, or mouth.

Contact your local doctor or emergency room if you notice any of the above symptoms.

_____
School nurse

_____
Telephone number

STUDENT EMERGENCY CARD

Date _____

School _____

Grade _____

Student's name _____

          Last   **First**   **Middle**

Birthdate _____

Address _____

Home telephone _____

City _____ Zip _____

To parent or guardian: To serve your child in case of accident or sudden illness, it is necessary that you furnish the following information for emergency calls:

Name	**Business address**	**Business telephone**
Mother		
Father		

List two neighbors or nearby relatives who will assume temporary care of your child if you cannot be reached:

Name _____ Name _____

Address _____ Tel. _____ Address _____ Tel. _____

Health information: List any health conditions such as heart disease, diabetes, epilepsy, severe allergies, eye or ear problems, any chronic condition, etc.

Explanation _____

_____

Doctor: Choice 1 _____ Choice 2 _____

      Telephone number _____ Telephone number _____

Hospital choice: Address _____ Telephone Number _____

IMPORTANT: Please complete reverse side of card.

(Back of Emergency Card)

I, the undersigned, do hereby authorize officials of _____ School District to contact directly the persons named on this card and do authorize the named physicians to render such treatment as may be deemed necessary in an emergency, for the health of said child.

In the event that physicians, other persons named on this card, or parents cannot be contacted, the school officials are hereby authorized to take whatever action is deemed necessary in their judgment, for the health of the aforesaid child.

I will not hold the school district financially responsible for the emergency care and/or transportation for said child.

_____

Signature of parent or guardian

_____

Student's last name   **First**   **Initial**

FORMS FOR
ADULT PERSONNEL

EMPLOYER'S FIRST REPORT OF INJURY OR ILLNESS

The Employer's First Report of Injury or Illness is used by many states in worker's compensation–related accidents. The details of this form vary from state to state. It may be filled out by school health personnel, administrative personnel, or the employee.

CERTIFICATE OF EXAMINATION OF SCHOOL
PERSONNEL FOR TUBERCULOSIS

If your state requires a freedom-of-tuberculosis certificate (skin text or X ray) as a condition of employment in the school district, use the following Certificate of Examination of School Personnel for Tuberculosis.

EMPLOYER'S FIRST REPORT OF INJURY OR ILLNESS

Instructions: Send copy to insurance carrier (name and address).

State's number	Board number _____
For:	File _____
	Carrier _____
	Employer _____

Carrier's file no. _____

OSHA file no.

(The spaces above are not to be completed by the employer.)

Employer

1. Name of employer _____ Telephone no. _____
2. Office address: No. and st. _____ City or town _____ State _____ Zip code _____
3. Insured by _____ Policy no. _____
4. Give nature of business (or article manufactured) _____

Time and Place

5. (a) Location of plant or place where accident occurred, no. and street { _____ City _____
   Did accident occur on employer's premises? ☐ Yes ☐ No. { County _____ State _____ Zip code _____
   Department where injured _____ Department regularly employed in _____
   (b) If injured in a mine, did accident occur on surface, underground, shaft, drill or mill? _____
   (c) Was employee hired or if a Texas resident, recruited in Texas? ☐ Yes ☐ No
   (d) If injury occurred out of Texas, on what date was employee transferred out of state? _____
6. Date of injury _____ 19 ____ Day of week _____ Hour of day _____ A.M. _____ P.M.
7. First day unable to labor _____ 19 ____ A.M. _____ P.M. 8. Was injured paid in full for this day? _____
9. When did you or supervisor first know of injury? _____ 10. Name of supervisor _____

Injured Person

                    Full first name   Middle initial   Last name
11. Name of injured _____ Social security no. _____
12. Address: no. and st. _____ City or town _____ State _____ Zip code _____
13. Telephone no. _____ Telephone no. friend or relative _____ Speak English ☐ Yes ☐ No
14. (a) Age ____ (b) Sex ____ (c) Marital status _____ (d) Minor children _____
15. (a) Occupation when injured _____ (b) Was this his or her regular occupation? _____
    (c) Under what classification code is employee's payroll reported to insurance carrier? _____
16. (a) How long employed by you _____ (b) Piece or time worker _____ (c) Wages per hour $ _____
17. (a) No. hours per day ____ (b) Wages per day $ ____ (c) No. days worked per week ____ (d) Average weekly earnings $ ____
    (e) If board, lodging, fuel, or other advantages were furnished in addition to wages, give estimated market value per day, week, or month ____
18. Was injured employee officer, director, partner, or owner? _____

Cause of Injury

19. Machine, tool or thing causing injury _____ 20. Kind of power (hand, foot, electrical, steam, etc.) _____
21. Part of machine on which accident occurred _____
22. (a) Name the safety appliance or regulation provided _____ (b) Was it in use at time? _____
23. Was accident caused by injured's failure to use or observe safety appliance or regulation? _____
24. Describe fully how accident occurred, and state what employee was doing when injured _____
25. Names and addresses of witnesses _____

Nature of Injury

26. Describe the injury or illness in detail and indicate the part of body affected _____
27. Probable length of disability _____ 28. Has injured returned to work? _____
    If so, date and hour _____ At what wage $ _____
29. At what occupation? _____
30. (a) Name of address of physician (if known) _____
    (b) Name and address of hospital (if known) _____

Fatal Cases

31. Has injured died? _____ If so, give date of death _____

Date of this report _____ Firm name _____

Employer's location no. _____ Report no. _____ Signed by _____ Official title _____

Industrial Accident Board requires completion of all applicable items on this form.

MEDICAL EVALUATION RECORD

Instructions: Board of Education policy requires each new employee to furnish evidence of a physical examination certified by a physician licensed by the   . This completed physical examination form must be submitted to your principal/department head the first day you report for duty.

Personal Information (please print).

Social security no. | | | | | | | | | | | Name |_____ |_____ |_____ |
                                                        Last   First   M

School _____   Location no. |_____ |

Race   1☐Anglo   2☐Black   3☐Mexican-American   4☐Native American   5☐Oriental
            6☐Other   (American Indian)

Sex   1☐Male   2☐Female   Birthdate _____   Date of exam _____

Address _____   Phone no. _____

Medical Information

	(1)	(2)	(3)
1. Do you think this employee will be able to perform his or her position throughout the next school year? If explanation needed, check box and explain on back.	☐ Yes	☐ No	☐ Explanation on back
2. History of medical problems? If explanation needed, check box and explain on back.	☐ No	☐ Yes	☐ Explanation on back
3. Current medical problems? If explanation needed, check box and explain on back.	☐ No	☐ Yes	☐ Explanation on back
4. Weight:	☐ Normal	☐ Excessively high	☐ Excessively low
5. Blood pressure.	☐ Normal	☐ High	☐ Low
6. Vision (with glasses if worn):	☐ 20/20	☐ 20/30–20/40	☐ 20/50 or worse
7. Hearing (audiogram if indicated):	☐ Normal	☐ Abnormal	
8. Urinalysis			
Sugar	☐ Not present	☐ Present	
Protein	☐ Not present	☐ Present	

Observations (Please check all categories.)

	Normal	Abnormal	Not Examined	Description
1. Eyes/ears	☐	☐	☐	_____
2. Nose/mouth/throat/neck	☐	☐	☐	_____
3. Lungs/chest/breast	☐	☐	☐	_____
4. Heart/vessels	☐	☐	☐	_____
5. Abdomen	☐	☐	☐	_____
6. Genitalia	☐	☐	☐	_____
7. Bones/joints/extremities	☐	☐	☐	_____
8. Neurological/reflexes	☐	☐	☐	_____
9. Skin/lymphatics	☐	☐	☐	_____

I certify that on this date I made the evaluations recorded above for this employee. In my opinion, he or she is in good mental and physical health, including freedom from communicable diseases, except as noted above.

                                                            D.O.
Date _____ Signed _____   M.D.   Telephone _____

Printed name _____   Address _____

State Board of Medical Examiners license no. _____

CERTIFICATE OF EXAMINATION
OF SCHOOL PERSONNEL FOR TUBERCULOSIS

This is to certify that _____, No. _____,

Name (first, middle, last)   (employee number)

was examined on _____ for the disease of tuberculosis and was found to (be free of) active

(have)

tuberculosis. The following were performed in connection with the examination:

Tuberculin test: Date _____   Result _____   **Negative reaction**

_____ **Not done**   _____   **Positive reaction**

Chest Xray: Date _____   Report _____ **Normal chest findings**

_____ **Not done**   _____ **Abnormal chest findings**

_____

Physician's signature

_____ **MD/DO license number** _____

(State)

14

LEAVE FORM FOR HEALTH AND/OR DISABILITY

Instructions: Sections I and II are to be completed at the time a leave for health or disability is requested. Section III should be completed only when the employee is ready to return to work.

Section I (To be completed by employee.)

1. Employee's name _____ Social security no. _____

2. Employee's job title _____ School _____

3. List names of all physicians consulted for this health problem and/or disability.

_____   _____
Physician's name   Telephone number

_____   _____
Physician's name   Telephone number

_____   _____
Physician's name   Telephone number

I hereby authorize any physician, hospital, insurance company, or employer to release any and all information regarding the medical history, diagnosis and treatment of my disability or illness. A copy of this authorization shall be valid as the original.

Signature of employee _____ Date _____

Section II (To be completed by physician or supplier of information.)

1. Date patient first consulted you for this condition _____

2. Diagnosis/nature of patient's illness, disability, or injury (if disability is pregnancy, proceed to entry no. 5). _____

_____

_____

3. Symptoms _____

_____

Has patient ever had same or similar symptoms? When? _____

4. Treatment prescribed, including length of treatment _____

_____

_____

5. Prognosis _____

6. Probable date of return to work _____

_____   _____
Physician's printed/typed name   Physician's signature

                                         _____
                                         Date

Individuals who are presently on leave and are ready to return to work must complete the back of this form.

RETURN TO WORK REQUEST FORM

I hereby request that my health/disability leave be terminated, and that I be placed back on active duty status. To the best of my knowledge, I am physically and emotionally capable of carrying out my full job reponsibilities.

_____   _____
Employee's signature   Date

Section III (To be completed by the physician when the patient is fully recovered and able to return to work.)

1. **Any remaining symptoms** _____

_____

2. **Continued treatment** _____

_____

3. **Prognosis** _____

_____

Instructions: Additional comments may be added in the space provided below.

I have discussed with my patient the advisability of his or her returning to work. He or she and I are fully aware of the responsibilities associated with the position and the physical and emotional stress that may accompany carrying out these job responsibilities. In my professional opinion _____ is fully recovered and will be able to assume all the responsibilities of his or her job on _____.

_____   _____
Physician's signature   Date

Comments _____

_____

Section IV (To be completed by school district physician, uncomplicated pregnancy excepted.)

_____ 1. I approve the employee's request to return to work.

_____ 2. Based on the available information, I am not able at this time to approve this request to return to work. I recommend a medical review before his or her request to return to work can be acted upon.

_____   _____
Physician's signature   Date

TRANSPORTATION DIVISION:
MEDICAL EXAMINATION REPORT FOR REGULAR AND/OR SUBSTITUTE SCHOOL BUS DRIVERS

Planned Use of Data: The screening of school bus driver applicants, and local school administration documentation that applicants meet all required medical and physiological requirements.

Instructions:

(1) Do not return completed form to applicant. The completed and signed form should be returned to the school and/or institution that is considering the employment of the applicant being examined.

(2) This form is to be completed by a physician who is duly registered and licensed to practice medicine.

(3) The applicant shall be disqualified for any of the physical or mental conditions listed on the back side of this form.

(4) The examining physician shall fill in all required information. (The use of check marks will not be allowed.)

Applicant's Information

Name _____ Age _____ Sex _____ Height _____ Weight _____

Address _____

Medical History

Applicant's medical history: Do you have or have you ever had

Diabetes	Yes ____ No ____	**Vision problem**	Yes ____ No ____
Tuberculosis	Yes ____ No ____	**Hearing problem**	Yes ____ No ____
Heart disease	Yes ____ No ____	**Asthma**	Yes ____ No ____
High blood pressure	Yes ____ No ____	**Dizziness or fainting spells**	Yes ____ No ____
Physical deformities	Yes ____ No ____	**Back injury**	Yes ____ No ____
Speech defect	Yes ____ No ____	**Hernia**	Yes ____ No ____
Head injury	Yes ____ No ____	**Other chronic diseases or defects**	Yes ____ No ____
Convulsions or epilepsy	Yes ____ No ____		
Alcoholism or drug addiction	Yes ____ No ____	**Nervous disorders or mental illness**	Yes ____ No ____
Syphilis	Yes ____ No ____		
		Do you take any medication or drugs to correct blood pressure or of a sedative nature	Yes ____ No ____

Comments _____

I certify that the above statements and/or information are correct to the best of my knowledge and belief.

_____   _____

Date   Applicant's signature

TRANSPORTATION DIVISION:
MEDICAL EXAMINATION REPORT FOR REGULAR AND/OR SUBSTITUTE SCHOOL BUS DRIVERS
Page 2

Note to Examining Physician: Please review the disqualification factors listed on the back page of this form. Fill in all required information, and abstain from the use of checkmarks in the listed blanks.

Appearance _____ Blood pressure _____

HEENT: Nose and throat _____

Eyes: OD _____ **OS** _____ **Snellen: OD 20/** _____ **OS 20/** _____ **Corrected: OD 20/** _____ **OS 20/** _____

     Peripheral vision in degrees: OD _____ **OS** _____ **Color vision** _____

     Pupillary reflex: OD _____ **OS** _____ **Muscle balance: OD** _____ **OS** _____

     Ears: R _____ **L** _____ **Hearing: Normal** _____ **Abnormal** _____

Lungs _____

Heart _____

Abdomen _____

Genitalia (evidence of venereal disease) _____

Hernia _____

Extremities _____

Spine _____

Neurological: Romberg _____ **Deep tendon reflexes** _____ **Coordination** _____

Skin _____

Laboratory: Urinalysis: Sugar _____ **Albumin** _____

Comment on abnormal findings _____

Physician's Certificate

I hereby certify that _____ has been examined by me in accordance with the medical examination report form above. The above-named applicant is qualified _____ disqualified _____ to perform the duties of a school bus driver in accordance with the disqualification factors governing this examination.

Qualified only while wearing glasses _____.

Qualified only while wearing hearing aid _____.

Address	Telephone	Date

Physician's signature

Return completed and signed form to
_____
County/district superintendent
_____
School address
_____
City   State   Zip

Physician's School Bus Driver Disqualification Sheet

The primary concern for any school bus driver is the safety and welfare of the children that ride his or her bus. In addition to the driving task, a school bus driver must be able to control the bus passengers and deal with any emergency or other situation that may arise.

The physician shall disqualify the applicant for the following physical or mental conditions.

I. Physical conditions
  A. Vision
    1. Eye diseases
      a. Eye diseases requiring the care of a physician,* exclude the fitting of lenses.
      b. Cannot readily distinguish red, green, or yellow.
      c. Has vision in only one eye or visual abnormalities that would impair his or her driving ability.
  B. Circulatory diseases
    1. Heart diseases
      a. Applicant has received coronary bypass surgery within a period of six (6) months
      b. Has had a heart attack within the past six (6) months, which has a severity rating of Class I of the American Heart Association's functional and therapeutic classification. Other classifications of attacks result in automatic disqualification.
    2. Hypertension
      a. Applicant has uncontrolled hypertension or is taking medication to correct high blood pressure that produces a sedative effect or other reactions that would impair mental or physical functions.
    3. Cerebral vascular disease (stroke, cerebral hemorrhage, or clots)
      a. Has had an alteration of consciousness with or without convulsions during the past 12 months
      b. Under the care of a physician
  C. Metabolic diseases
    1. Diabetes
      a. Is taking insulin.
      b. Has "blacked out" or lost consciousness during the past 12 months.
  D. Respiratory
    1. Respiratory diseases
      a. Confirmed shortness of breath or audible wheezing that would affect safe driving abilities.
  E. Physical impairment
    1. Physical
      a. Has loss of any of the extremities (hand, arm, foot, or leg) as stated in the Motor Carrier Safety Regulations of Federal Highway Administration 49 CFR 391.
      b. Stiffness of joints from arthritis or other conditions that would impair applicant's ability to drive a bus or react to emergency situations.
    2. Voice
      a. Has speech defect that would make it impossible to give clear directions or commands.
    3. Hearing
      a. Applicant's hearing is not a minimum of 10/15 by whispered voice. Hearing aid is permissible.
II. Mental or emotional disorders
  A. Mental or emotional
    1. Neurological disorders
      a. Applicant has a history of recurring seizures or has experienced a seizure within the past two years.
    2. Mental disorders
      a. Any known mental disorder that would impair driving ability or create an unsatisfactory association with children.
    3. Drug and/or alcohol abuse
      a. Is currently addicted to the use of drugs or alcohol
      b. Applicant has demonstrated abusive use of alcohol and/or drugs within the past 24 months.
      c. Any applicant with a history of drug and/or alcohol abuse shall be reevaluated annually prior to the beginning of employment.

*"Under the care of a physician" is defined as having been referred to for treatment or having received treatment from a physician for the medical condition(s) indicated in the past 12 months without a release from further treatment.

FORMS FOR ATHLETICS AND PHYSICAL EDUCATION

PHYSICAL EXAMINATIONS

All states and/or state education agencies have regulations governing health evaluations prior to participation in athletic competition. The type and detail of the examination and the professional qualifications of the individual performing the evaluation vary. In most states, the signature of a licensed physician is required. In a few states, the type and frequency of the examination is left to the discretion of the local school district.

Many sports medicine specialists emphasize that a "sports directed" medical history is more important than the traditional hands-on physical exam. Also, the physical exam should be directed at discovering brain, bone, muscle, tendon, and joint weaknesses that predispose an athlete to injury. The condition of such items as the tonsils is of lesser importance.

The frequency of the health evaluation varies also. Most states require an annual hands-on physical exam with no health history. Some states (ten in 1982) require a complete history and physical evaluation once or twice in the athlete's school career, with only an annual update of the history if there have been no problems since the last exam. (This last arrangement is recommended by several sports medicine specialists and is favored by the author.)

MEDICAL EXCUSE FROM PHYSICAL EDUCATION

The Medical Excuse from Physical Education is an important, frequently used, form in most schools. Filled out by a conscientious doctor, it can be most helpful for excusing from physical education those children who have legitimate medical reasons for not exercising because it will aggravate their illness. However, some physicians merely send a hastily scrawled note on a prescription pad asking that the student be excused from physical education for the entire school year for minor or frivolous reasons. This is often done in response to pressure from the parents.

Since physical education is a required course in many jurisdictions, and since some students, especially obese students, do not like to participate in physical education, the school nurse or a school medical consultant is often helpful in mediating disputes.

ADAPTED PHYSICAL EDUCATION RECOMMENDATIONS

Adapted physical education may be required for permanent conditions such as cerebral palsy, heart disease, muscle diseases, or other long-term disorders. Temporary adapted physical education may be necessary for sprains, strains, convalescence from a long-term illness, or other disorders that leave the student weak and out of condition.

ATHLETIC DEPARTMENT

Home address _____ Telephone _____

1. Has had injuries requiring medical attention?	Yes	No
2. Has had illness lasting more than a week?	Yes	No
3. Is under a physician's care now?	Yes	No
4. Takes medication now?	Yes	No
5. Wears glasses?	Yes	No
Contact lenses?	Yes	No
6. Has had a surgical operation?	Yes	No
7. Has been in a hospital (except for tonsillectomy)?	Yes	No
8. Do you know of any reason why this individual should not participate in all sports?	Yes	No
9. Have you ever been knocked out or had a concussion?	Yes	No
10. Are you allergic to any medicines?	Yes	No
(examples: aspirin, Tylenol)		
11. Are you missing any paired organs?	Yes	No
(examples: eyes, ears, kidneys, testicles)		
12. Do you wear any dental appliance such as a crown, bridge, partial, or full plate?	Yes	No
13. Most recent tetanus toxoid _____. Booster required only every ten years.	Yes	No

Date

Please explain any "Yes" answers to the above questions:

_____

_____

_____

Student Participation

_____ _____ _____ _____

First name   **Last name**   **Middle initial**   **School**   **Date**   **Date of birth**

This application to compete in interscholastic athletics for the school year _____ for the above high school is entirely voluntary on my part and is made with the understanding that I have not violated any of the eligibility rules and regulations of the state association.

_____

Signature of student

Parental Approval

*I hereby give my consent for the above-named student (1) to represent his or her school for the school year _____ in athletic activities except those crossed out on this form by the examining physician, provided that such athletic activities are approved by the state association: (2) to accompany any school team of which he or she is a member on any of its local or out-of-town trips. I authorize the school to obtain, through a physician of its own choice, any emergency medical care that may become reasonably necessary for the student in the course of such athletic activities or such travel. I also agree not to hold the school or anyone acting in its behalf responsible for any injury occurring to the above-named student in the course of such athletic activities or such travel."

_____   _____

Typed or printed name of parent or guardian   Signature of parent or guardian

_____   _____

Date   Address

Name of health/accident/hospitalization insurance _____

These medical forms are adapted from the *American Medical Association Handbook,* "Medical Evaluation of the Athlete," which can be obtained from the American Medical Association. It is suggested that team physicians acquaint themselves with the above handbook.

ATHLETIC DEPARTMENT
Page 2

Physical Examination*

Weight _____ **Height** _____ **Pulse** _____ **B/P** _____

Eyes _____ **Ears** _____ **Nose** _____

Teeth _____ **Lungs** _____ **Throat** _____

Heart _____ **Liver** _____ **Spleen** _____

Neurological _____ **Musculoskeletal** _____ **Genitalia** _____

Hernia _____ **Feet** _____ **Spine** _____

*√ normal; x, abnormal; NE, not examined.

Comments on any abnormal findings _____

_____

_____

_____

_____

Optional at discretion of examining physician:

Hemaglobin or hematocrit _____

Urinalysis _____

Vision _____ **Hearing** _____

I certify that I have on this date examined this student and that, on the basis of the examination requested by the school authorities and the student's medical history as furnished to me, I have found no reason that would make it medically inadvisable for this student to compete in supervised athletic activities, *except those crossed out below.*

Baseball	Football	Rowing	Softball	Track
Basketball	Hockey	Skating	Speedball	Volleyball
Cross-country	Golf	Skiing	Swimming	Wrestling (estimated desirable
Field hockey	Gymnastics	Soccer	Tennis	weight level ____ pounds)

Date of examination _____

_____
Printed or typed name of examining physician

Physician's address _____

_____
Signature of examining physician

If an athlete transfers to another school, this form—both sides—should accompany him or her.

24

FITNESS CHECKUP RECORD AND PARENTAL APPROVAL
FOR PARTICIPATION IN HIGH SCHOOL ATHLETICS

Name _____

Address _____

City or town _____ State _____

Name of school _____

In case of emergency, notify

Name _____ Relationship: Parent ☐   Guardian ☐

Address _____

Home phone _____ Other phone _____

Note to parents: Please
   Fill out this page carefully.
   Have your son or daughter take it to examining physician.
   Follow the doctor's advice about limitations.

Health History

Has had (check if "yes")

Head or brain injury	☐	Heart condition or heart disease	☐
Unconsciousness	☐	Poliomyelitis	☐
Sprains of any joints	☐	Rheumatic fever	☐
Broken bones	☐	Diabetes	☐
Serious eye trouble	☐	Allergy to any medication	☐
Kidney injuries	☐	Hernia	☐

Date of last tetanus immunization _____

Describe _____

_____

_____

Check here if none of above applies ☐

Have ever been (check if "yes")
   Treated for by a doctor?   ☐
   Operated on?   ☐
   Admitted to hospital?   ☐

Explain _____

Parental or Guardian's Permission

I hereby give my consent for the above student to engage in approved high school athletics and also agree that the above statements of medical history are accurate. I also give permission to give tetanus immunizations when available.

Date _____ Signed _____
                                                        Parent or guardian

FITNESS CHECKUP RECORD AND PARENTAL APPROVAL
FOR PARTICIPATION IN HIGH SCHOOL ATHLETICS
Page 2

Suggested Physical Examination Form for Athletic Participation

To be filled out by examining physician:

Name of student _____ **Height** _____ **Weight** _____ **Age** _____

Body development (circle number)   10 9 8 7 6 5 4 3 2 1
                                               (Heavy)   (Medium)   (Slender)

Examination

	Satisfactory	Unsatisfactory	Explanation if unsatisfactory
Teeth	☐	☐	
Extremities	☐	☐	
Heart	☐	☐	
Hernia	☐	☐	
Other	☐	☐	
_____	☐	☐	
_____	☐	☐	
_____	☐	☐	

Special defects _____

Recommendations for athletic participation _____

_____

_____

Date examined _____ **19_____ By** _____
                                                          Physician licensed to practice medicine

This medical record belongs either in the high school office or in the school physicians records whichever will be most beneficial in time of an emergency.

Record During School Year

Date	Injury	How injury was obtained?	Treatment	Date of return to competition

PARENT'S PERMIT AND HEALTH QUESTIONNAIRE

Instructions: This form must be completed, signed, and returned to the school each year before the student will be permitted to practice or play.

Name of student _____   Birthdate _____
                          (Type or print)   Month   Date   Year

High school _____   Grade in school ___ 9 - 10 - 11 - 12 ___
                                                                        (circle one)

      State High School League regulations provide that any student who intends to participate in high school interscholastic athletics and cheerleading activities must have on file in this school a record of a satisfactory physical examination performed by a physician within the previous three years. More frequent examinations may be required. The student named above has this record on file. _____ Yes _____ No

The following questions must be answered by the parent or guardian:

	Please circle
1. Has the student been hospitalized since the above physical examination?	Yes No
2. Has the student had a major injury since the above physical examination?	Yes No
3. Has the student been found to have only one organ of usually paired organs? (example: only one kidney or one good eye)	Yes No
4. Has the student required medication on a daily or episodic routine? (example: insulin daily or asthma medication with an attack)	Yes No
5. Has the student been knocked unconscious at any time within the past 12 months?	Yes No
6. Does the student require a tetanus (lockjaw) booster? (needed every 10 years)	Yes No
7. Do you know of or believe there is any health reason why this student should not participate in interscholastic athletics or cheerleading activities?	Yes No

      If so, why? _____

_____

The undersigned, herewith,

1. Grants the above-named student permission to participate in all league activities.
2. Grants permission to take the student on supervised trips connected with league activities.
3. Understands that the student must refrain from practice or play during medical treatment until he or she is discharged from treatment or is given a written permit by the attending physician to resume participation.
4. Certifies that the answers to the questions above are correct and true.

Date _____   Signed _____
            Month, day, and year   Signature of parent or guardian

Parent's permit and health questionnaire must be completed, signed, and placed on file in the school office each year before the student will be permitted to practice or play.

STUDENT-PARENT-PHYSICIAN'S CERTIFICATE

Instructions: Detach; to be retained by student or parent.

Individual Eligibility Rules (grades 9 through 12)

Attention, athlete: **Your school is a member of the** _____ **and follows established rules. To be eligible to represent your school in interschool athletics** *you*

1. **Must be a regular bona fide student in good standing in the school you represent.**
2. **Must have enrolled not later than the fifteenth day of the current semester.**
3. **Must have received passing grades in at least four full-credit subjects or the equivalent during your last grading period except that the semester grades shall take precedence at the end of a semester and must be currently passing in at least four full credit subjects or the equivalent.**
4. **Must not have reached your nineteenth birthday before August 15 (September 1, beginning 19) preceding the current school year.**
5. **Must have been enrolled in your present high school last semester or at a junior high school from which your high school receives its students.**
   Unless you are entering the ninth grade for the first time.
   Unless you are transferring from a school district or territory with a corresponding bona fide move on the part of your parents.
   Unless your former school is nonaccredited, was a correctional school, was discontinued or consolidated, and you were required to transfer to your present school.
   Unless you are legally adopted, are a foreign exchange student under a full-year program, are under the direction of an orphanage or State Department of Welfare, are required to change residence by court order, or are a ward of a guardian who resides in your new school district or territory, have not participated in a high school varsity contest, are married and established residence in a new district or territory, or are over 18 years of age and principal of former school approves.
   Unless you are transferring for the first time from one public school to another by desegregation directive.
   Note: **You must have been eligible in the school from which you transferred.**
6. **Must not have been enrolled more than four fall semesters and four spring semesters beginning with grade 9, or have represented a high school in a sport more than four years.**
7. **Must be an amateur (... have not participated under an assumed name; have not accepted money or merchandise directly or indirectly for athletic participation; have not accepted awards, gifts, or honors from colleges or their alumni; have not signed a professional contract.)**
8. **Must have filed with your principal each school year, between May 1 and your first practice, your completed Student-Parent-Physician certificate.**
9. **Must not have transferred from one school to another for athletic purposes as a result of undue influence or persuasion by any person or group.**
10. **Must not have received, in recognition of your athletic ability, any award not approved by your principal.**
11. **Must not accept commercial awards that advertise any business firm or individuals or awards designating "All-State" or "All-American" status.**
12. **Must not participate in an athletic contest during the authorized contest season for that sport as an individual or on any team other than their school team. (Participation in football or boys' basketball before or after the authorized contest season causes ineligibility for a period not to exceed 365 days.)**
13. **Must not reflect discredit upon your school or create a disruptive influence on the discipline, good order, or moral or educational environment in your school.**
14. **Must not participate out of season in an organized boys' basketball or football practice, game, demonstration, exhibition, or scrimmage. Limited participation is permitted in basketball and/or football camps approved by** _____.
15. **Must not participate in a tryout, demonstration, or audition as a prospective college athlete. Seniors may participate in such after end of season of that sport. Girls may participate in auditions under certain conditions. Consult your high school principal.**
16. **Must not participate with or against a student enrolled below grade 9.**
17. **Must not, while on a grade 9 junior high team, participate with or against a student enrolled in grade 11 or 12.**
18. **Must, if absent five or more days due to illness or injury, present to your principal written verification from a licensed physician stating that you may participate again.**
19. **Must not participate in specialized camps, clinics, or schools for more than 14 nonschool out-of-season calendar days per sport per year.**
20. **This is only a summary of the rules. Contact your school officials for further information and before participating outside your school.**

Name_____ School _____ School yr _____
    Last (print)   First   Initial

Grade_____Date of birth _____Age_____(check one) Female_____Male_____

Address_____Phone_____

With whom do you live? (Check one.) Parent_____Guardian_____Other_____

School attended last semester _____

STUDENT-PARENT-PHYSICIAN'S CERTIFICATE
Page 2

Part I—Student Certificate (to be signed by student)

I have read the attached condensed eligibility rules of the _____ High School Athletic Association and believe I am eligible to represent my present school in athletics. If accepted as a representative, I agree to abide by said rules and regulations of my school. To the best of my knowledge I have suffered no injury or illness in the past that would hinder my participation in my chosen sport(s).

Date _____ Student signature _____

Part II—Parent Consent (To be completed and signed by parent or guardian.)

In accordance with the rules, I hereby give my consent for the above-named student to participate in the following interschool sports *not marked out:*

Boy's Sports: Baseball, basketball, cross-country, football, golf, gymnastics, swimming, tennis, track, wrestling.

Girl's Sports: Basketball, cross-country, golf, gymnastics, softball, swimming, tennis, track, volleyball.

I understand that participation may necessitate travel and early dismissal from classes. *Please check appropriate space:* He or she has school student accident insurance (   ), has football insurance through the school (   ), has adequate family insurance coverage (   ).

Date _____ Parent-guardian signature _____

Part III—Student Medical History (To be completed by parent or family physician.)

Name of student _____
Parent's name _____ Phone _____

(Circle one.)

Yes No	1.	Has had injuries requiring medical attention.
Yes No	2.	Has had illness lasting more than a week.
Yes No	3.	Is under physician's care now.
Yes No	4.	Takes medication now.
Yes No	5.	Wears glasses. Contact lenses Yes No
Yes No	6.	Has had a surgical operation.
Yes No	7.	Has been in hospital (except for tonsillectomy)
Yes No	8.	Do you know of any reason why the individual should not participate in all sports?

Please explain any "Yes" answers to above questions.

_____
_____

Yes No	9.	Has had complete poliomyelitis immunization.
Yes No	10.	Has had a dental checkup within the past six months.
Yes No	11.	Most recent tetanus toxoid immunization date _____

Parent or physician's signature _____

Part IV—Physician's Certificate (To be completed annually by physician holding unlimited license to practice medicine.)

Name of student _____ School _____
Significant past illness or injury _____
Grade _____ Age _____ Height _____ Weight _____ Blood pressure _____

Examination	Satis.	Unsatis.	Not examined	Examination	Satis.	Unsatis.	Not examined
Vision				Musculoskeletal			
Hearing				Skin			
Respiratory				Neurological			
Cardiovascular				Lab Tests—urinalysis			
Liver, spleen, kidney				Other			
Hernia, genitalia							

I certify that I have examined this student as indicated and find him or her physically able to compete in supervised athletics *not marked out:*
Boy's Sports: Baseball, basketball, cross-country, football, golf, gymnastics, swimming, tennis, track, wrestling.*
Girl's Sports: Basketball, cross-country, golf, gymnastics, softball, swimming, tennis, track, volleyball.
*Weight loss permitted to make lower weight class in wrestling? Yes _____ No _____ If Yes may lose _____ pounds.
Physicians address _____ Phone _____
Date of examination/certification _____ Signed _____ M.D.

MEDICAL WAIVER FOR ATHLETIC PARTICIPATION

Parental Notification

Name _____ School _____

During the routine preparticipation athletic physical on _____ the following
Date

condition(s) was discovered.

1. _____ 2. _____

Because of the increased possibility of athletic injury, it will be necessary for him or her to have a further medical evaluation before he or she can participate in the athletic program.

Approved _____ _____
School principal   Athletic trainer or school nurse

Physician's Report

I have examined _____ on _____
Date

and recommend that he or she be *allowed—not allowed* to participate in the athletic program as follows.
(Circle one)

1. No limitation   **2. Participate only under following conditions:**

_____

_____

_____
Physician's printed name

_____
Physician's signature

Parental Waiver

I, the parent or legal guardian of _____,
Name of athlete

have been informed of the disqualifying conditions discovered during the above medical evaluation and that he or she is at increased risk for further and possible serious injury.

Despite the conditions described above, I hereby give consent for my son or daughter to participate in the following sports:

1. _____ 2. _____ 3. _____ 4. _____

I also agree to hold the   School District harmless in case of injury.

_____
Printed name of parent or legal guardian

_____
Signature of parent or legal guardian

MEDICAL EXCUSE FROM PHYSICAL EDUCATION

Name _____

Address _____ School _____

Dear Doctor:

We have received a request that your patient be excused from physical exercise while at school. Physical Education is a course required by state law, and continued absence will result in loss of credit for this course.

Will you please help us to place this student properly by filling in the form below?

Activities (Cross out activities not considered appropriate for pupil.)

Archery	Golf	Running games	Volleyball
Badminton	Gymnastics	Shuffleboard	Walking
Basketball	Handball	Softball	Weight lifting
Bowling	Horseshoe	Soccer	Wrestling
Calisthenics	pitching	Tennis	Others (specify)
Dance	Jogging	Track and field	_____
Fitness testing	Rope jumping	Tumbling	_____
Football (touch)	Ping pong	Twelve-minute run/walk	_____

Nature of disability and reason for restriction _____

_____

_____

Duration of excuse _____

_____

Other suggested activities _____

_____

_____   _____
Printed name of doctor   Signature of doctor

_____   _____
Phone number   Date

31

ADAPTED PHYSICAL EDUCATION RECOMMENDATIONS

Name _____   Birthdate _____

Address _____   Phone _____

School _____ Teacher _____ Grade _____

Instructions: To be filled out by the physician.

Diagnosis or description of the condition _____

_____

_____

Condition: Permanent _____ Temporary _____

If temporary, may return to unrestricted activity _____.

                                                                        Date

Functional Restrictions

Pupil's condition is such that the intensity and type of activity should be limited. He or she is capable of participating to the extent of

_____ Unrestricted physical activity.

_____ No competitive sports; in other activities, should stop short of excessive fatigue or undue stress.

_____ No contact sports; other activity allowed.

_____ Moderate exercise with all running, jumping, and gymnastics excluded.

_____ Minimal activity; training in coordination only. Simple nonstrenuous activity (e.g., archery, Ping Pong).

_____ Recommend the following exercise: _____

_____

Musculoskeletal Restrictions

_____ Avoid activities involving upper extremities.

_____ Avoid activities involving neck, back, or abdomen.

_____ Avoid activities involving the lower extremities.

Comments _____

_____

Please call me if there are any questions about these restrictions.

Date _____ Signed _____ M.D.

PHYSICAL EDUCATION RESTRICTIONS

Name _____

Condition _____

The following P.E. restrictions are recommended:

_____ Regular program   _____ No P.E.

_____ After-school sports   _____ No contact sports

_____ No running   _____ No gymnastics

_____ No dressing   _____ No showers

Restricted activity _____

_____

Time limit: Days, beginning _____

               Weeks, beginning _____

               This semester _____

               Requested by: _____ Parent _____ Physician _____ Nurse

_____   _____
     Date   School nurse

FORMS FOR
CHILD ABUSE

All states require that child abuse be reported. The following forms allow the school nurse to record the pertinent background facts and describe any visible physical findings that may help the investigating authorities. If no physical assessment is done at school, as in most cases of sexual abuse, the nurse should record "no physical assessment performed."

For legal protection, it is wise to record the date and to whom reported. Each state has slightly different reporting requirements, so local statutes must be adhered to in adapting a form for use by each school district.

The three forms of child abuse you may encounter are:

1. Sexual abuse.
2. Emotional abuse and neglect.
3. Physical abuse.

SEXUAL ABUSE

It is not wise to attempt an examination of a sexually abused child at school. This is an extremely complicated issue, should only be done once, and should be done by those aware of all medical, emotional, social, and legal implications.

EMOTIONAL ABUSE AND NEGLECT

Emotional abuse and child neglect are difficult for school authorities to deal with. Definitions are highly variable and the Department of Human Services (DHS) case workers have high caseloads they are unable to investigate. School nurses and principals often try to deal with cases of this nature "in house" by supplying clothing, nurture, or food. Flagrant cases must, of course, be reported; if case workers do not investigate, a phone call to a DHS supervisor may help.

PHYSICAL ABUSE

Bruises should be described according to (1) location; (2) size—actual measurement in inches or centimeters; (3) color—red, blue, purple, green, yellow, brown; and (4) shape and general appearance.

For example:

There is a bruise on the outer part of the left thigh, 4 inches above the knee. It is about $1\frac{1}{2}'' \times 2''$ in size, purple and green in color, and irregular in shape (resembles the shape of a belt buckle).

NOTE: Because of legal implications—court appearances, depositions, lawsuits, and so on—most school administrators prefer that child abuse forms be filled out by nursing and educational professionals. If the form is completed by paraprofessionals, have it done jointly with a teacher or principal and have both sign it.

SUSPECTED CHILD ABUSE NURSING EVALUATION REPORTING FORM

Instructions: Distribute one copy to the principal and one to the Health Office and retain one for your records.

School _____

Name of student _____ D.O.B. _____

Address _____

Home or nearest telephone number _____

Name of parent or legal guardian _____

Relationship _____

Nature of suspected abuse: ☐ **Physical** ☐ **Sexual** ☐ **Emotional** ☐ **Neglect**
(Check appropriate box(es).)

Pertinent history _____

_____

_____

_____

_____

Findings on physical assessment _____

_____

_____

_____

_____

_____

_____

_____   _____
Date reported   **Agency reported to**

_____
Name and title of person reported to

_____   _____
Nurse's signature   **Date**

REPORT OF CHILD ABUSE OR NEGLECT

It's the law: Any person who believes that a child's physical or mental health or welfare has been or may be adversely affected by abuse or neglect, or that a child has died of abuse or neglect, must report his or her suspicions to the Department of Human Services and to a law enforcement agency.

An oral report must be made immediately to the nearest office of Child Protective Services, Department of Human Services, or to the 24-hour Child Abuse Hotline (1-800-252-5400), and to a local law enforcement agency. A written report must be made within five days.

Immunity: A person who, without malice, makes a report or suspected child abuse or neglect is immune from civil or criminal liability.

Confidentiality: Reports of child abuse or neglect are confidential. Information in the reports, including the name of the person who makes the report, may be used only for purposes consistent with the investigation of abuse or neglect.

Failure to report suspected physical or mental abuse or neglect of a child is a crime punishable by fine, imprisonment, or both.

(This form is furnished to help comply with the law.)

Detach, seal, and mail

Report of Child Abuse or Neglect

Name of child	Date of birth of age of child	Today's date
Child's home address (street, city, state, zip)		
Names of parents or persons responsible for child	**Relationship to child**	

Does the child have any brothers or sisters? ☐ Yes ☐ No ☐ Don't know

When and where can the child be seen? (give dates and places) _____

Type of Child Abuse or Neglect

☐ Burning ☐ Beating ☐ Fracture ☐ Sexual abuse ☐ Abandonment ☐ Malnutrition ☐ Internal injuries

☐ Physical neglect ☐ Medical neglect ☐ Lack of supervision ☐ Other (specify) _____

Briefly describe the situation and/or condition of the child _____

_____

Has this report already been called in? ☐ Yes, to local Child Protective Services ☐ Yes, to Child Abuse Hotline ☐ No

If yes, date _____ To whom? _____

Person Making This Report (Anonymous reports are accepted, but DHR staff will be able to do a better investigation if they can contact you.)

Name	Place of employment
Work address (street, city, state, zip)	**Work telephone no.**
Home address (street, city, state, zip) Or, I prefer to be contacted at home:	**Home telephone no.**

SUSPECTED CHILD ABUSE/NEGLECT

To: Child Protective Services

Student's name _____ Date of birth _____ Sex _____

Address _____

Name of parents or guardians _____

School _____ Grade _____ Matrix # _____

Description of injury (use reverse side of form if necessary):

Symbols:

- **A** Abrasion
- **Bl** Blister
- **Bu** Burn
- **Br** Bruise
- **La** Laceration
- **Le** Lesions
- **S** Scar
- **R** Rash
- **V** Vermin
- **O** Other (describe)

Severity

Mild (1)
Moderate (2)
Severe (3)

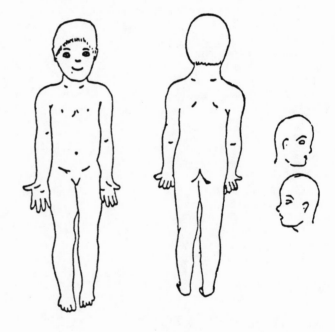

Signature and title of person making report _____ Date _____

To whom reported _____ Date of oral report _____

Copy filed in school nurse office.

FORMS FOR COMMUNICABLE DISEASE

PARENT NOTIFICATION

Districts must balance the value of notifying parents that their child has been exposed to a communicable disease against unduly alarming them. A medical consultant is invaluable in helping with this decision. Exposure to various illnesses require notices only be sent to parents of one specific class, athletes on the same team, and occasionally the entire student body.

Some of the diseases for which parents are notified are:

Hepatitis   Rabies exposure

Meningitis   Scabies

Impetigo   Lice (pediculosis)

Strep throat

Now that AIDS is being identified in some school children, districts are going to be faced with this difficult dilemma until it has been settled by the courts.

NURSE'S REPORT OF COMMUNICABLE DISEASE

Local health departments publish lists of reportable diseases:

1. Those that must be reported individually (hepatitis, syphilis, and so on)
2. Those reported by number of cases only (pediculosis, scabies, and so on)
3. Information about clusters of illnesses of unknown cause

School staff should report individual illnesses or clusters of cases to the school nurse or health aide for proper reporting to the health department.

School nurses are cautioned not to diagnose. However, health departments need to know about communicable diseases as early as possible. Depending on the nature of the condition, if early reporting is warranted, a disease can be reported as "suspect" or "tentative diagnosis . . ." until laboratory confirmation and/or physician's diagnosis can be obtained.

Hepatitis, differentiation between type A and type B, poses a common dilemma. Both diseases present the same type of onset, signs, and symptoms in most children. The usual blood tests that measure level of jaundice and liver function show the same results for both types. The blood tests (serum antibody profiles) that distinguish one from the other are expensive and may not be available for several days. For complete accuracy, the report to the health department (such as the Nurse's Report of Communicable Disease) should contain the name of the blood test upon which the diagnosis was based.

COMMUNICABLE DISEASE CHART

The Communicable Disease Chart was developed by one state health department to help guide the school nurse and/or delegated personnel. It is usually posted in a prominent place so as to help reinforce school personnel's action in communicable disease control.

All state health departments have published guidelines of this nature. Most states have legal reporting requirements that schools are mandated to follow.

The instructions for management of each case and school exclusion are usually not legal requirements. They are suggested guidelines, although some are debated. Some examples of these debated guidelines from the chart are:

1. *Common cold:* "school exclusion until clinical recovery." This is rarely necessary.
2. *Chicken pox:* "school exclusion until six days after last crop of blisters." Most infectious disease authorities feel that chicken pox is noncontagious five days after *onset* of fever or *first* blister.
3. *Pink eye:* "exclude until released by physician." Many cases of pink eye are either mildly or not at all contagious and need not be excluded.

HEPATITIS INFORMATION LETTER
(English)

Dear Parent:

A case of hepatitis has occurred in your child's classroom. We have taken the precautionary measures prescribed by the public health authorities to prevent the spread of the disease.

For your information, we would like to tell you what the American Academy of Pediatrics says about hepatitis. "It is a disease that is not very contagious (compared to measles, etc.) and therefore it is unusual for two cases to occur in the same classroom. It is usually mild in children. It is caused by a virus or germ that may be found in secretions of the mouth and nose, but is especially found in the urine and stool of the person with the disease. Therefore washing the hands after going to the bathroom is especially important.

"Protection with gamma globulin is recommended only for certain household contacts and people living in institutions such as orphanages or state hospitals."

If you have reason to believe that your child was exposed more intimately (spending the night at the home of the sick child, best friend, etc.) or if you have any other doubts or special questions, please call your family physician or contact the school nurse.

_____

School

HEPATITIS INFORMATION LETTER
(Spanish)

Apreciable padre de familia:

Un caso de hepatitis ha ocurrido en el salón de clase de su niño. Hemos tomado los medios de precaución prescritos por las autoridades de salubridad pública para prevenir el desarrollo de dicha enfermedad.

Para información suya, quisiéramos darle a saber lo que la Academia Americana de Pediatría dice acerca de la hepatitis. "Es una enfermedad no muy contagiosa (en comparación al sarampión, etc.) y por consiguiente es raro que ocurran dos casos en un mismo salón de clase. Generalmente es leve en los niños. Es causada por el virus que se puede encontrar en la secreción de la boca y la nariz, pero especialmente se halla en la orina y en el excremento de la persona con la enfermedad. Por esta razón es de suma importancia el lavarse las manos después de ir al baño.

"Se recomienda inyectarse con gamma globulina únicamente en caso de contactos entre la familia viviendo en la casa y si las personas viven en instituciones tales como orfanatorios, asilos, etc."

Si usted tiene motivo para creer que su niño fue expuesto más íntimamente (posiblemente haya pasado la noche en casa del niño enfermo o sea su mejor amigo) o si usted tiene cualesquier otra clase de duda o preguntas particulares, favor de llamar a su médico o de comunicarse con la enfermera de la escuela.

_____

Escuela

MENINGOCOCCAL MENINGITIS PARENT LETTER
(English)

Date _____

To the Parents:

One of the children in your child's class went home from school ill and was later diagnosed as having meningococcal meningitis. We suggest that you contact your family doctor for his recommendation.

_____
Principal

_____
School

MENINGOCOCCAL MENINGITIS PARENT LETTER
(Spanish)

Fecha _____

Para los Padres:

Uno de los niños en la clase de su hijo(a) resulto enfermo y fue diagnosticado que tenia la meningococcal meningitis. Sugerimos que se ponga usted en contacto con su doctor para su recomendación.

_____
Principal

_____
Escuela

EVIDENCE OF HEAD LICE

_____
Date

To the Parents of _____

You child's hair was examined at school today and found to have nits (eggs). This is a sign of head lice. Your child may not return to school until the hair has been washed with a medicated shampoo.

For your child to remain free of head lice, all household members should use this shampoo. Clothing, towels, bedlinen, combs and brushes should be washed in hot soapy water. Complete instructions are provided with the medicated shampoo.

Your child may not be readmitted to school until

      1. Medicated shampoo has been used.
      2. You have signed the form below and returned it to school.

_____
Principal

_____
Detach here and return

Parent Statement

I have shampooed my child _____ hair
                                                 Child's name
with medicated shampoo sent home from school or medicated shampoo from my physician.

Please readmit him/her to class.

_____
Parent

HEAD LICE INFORMATION LETTER

Dear Parents,

Head lice is a widely misunderstood "nuisance-type" health problem. Head lice can happen to anyone. It is not a sign of poor health habits or being dirty. Head lice can occur at any age, in any ethnic group, and to either sex. It doesn't just happen to "other people." It could happen to your children. So let's learn how to recognize a head lice infestation, how to treat it, and how to prevent it from happening again.

Head lice are tiny insects that live in human hair. They hatch from small eggs, called nits, that are attached to the base of individual hairs. The eggs hatch in about ten days, with the new lice reaching maturity in about two weeks. Since head lice multiply rapidly, they should be treated promptly.

Head lice can be transmitted in several ways—by playing "head to head" or by sharing personal items such as combs, hairbrushes, hats, ribbons, scarves, or other head coverings. It is important to remind your children of the reasons for not sharing these items. Personal cleanliness does *not* prevent a person from getting head lice.

What signs should you look for? Persistent itching of the head and back of the neck can indicate head lice. You should also look for infected scratch marks or a rash on the scalp. *Most important of all* look for nits attached to individual hairs. Sometimes, small white specks in the hair such as dandruff can be confused with nits. Nits, however, are very difficult to remove, while dandruff will brush away easily.

Instructions for Treatment and Control of Head Lice and Nits

1. Use a pediculicide such as Kwell (prescription only) or RID (nonprescription). *Follow directions on the bottle exactly.* (The Health Department supplies Kwell at no cost.)
2. After using the pediculicide, a vinegar rinse may help to loosen the nits.
3. Nit removal is *never easy,* but a special Derbac comb will help. This comb may be purchased at the pharmacy or is available through School Health Services for a $3.00 deposit. *Check especially at the nape of the neck, above the ears, and under bangs.*
4. Household disinfection should be carried out at the same time as the child's treatment. The Health Department does not recommend pediculicide spraying of rooms, rugs, etc.
   a. Soak combs and brushes for 10 minutes in a pediculicide.
   b. Wash bedding and clothing in very hot water. Dry 20 minutes in a hot dryer, or press with a hot iron.
   c. Nonwashable items such as pillows, blankets, stuffed animals, caps, and jackets should be dry cleaned, sealed in plastic bags for 20 days, or placed in a hot dryer for 20 minutes.
   d. Vacuum upholstered furniture and mattresses. Run a warm iron next to the cording on mattresses and cushions (check material for safe temperature).
5. Repeat treatment of the hair in 10 days to assure that if any nits have hatched, the lice will be killed before they can lay more eggs.

Please check children frequently and treat them immediately after learning they have lice. *No* child excluded for lice will be readmitted until *all lice and nits have been removed.*

Thank you for your cooperation. If you have any questions, please call your school nurse.

PEDICULOSIS INFORMATION LETTER
(English)

Dear Parent:

Each year many children are found to have lice. Sometimes they are discovered by the teacher, sometimes by the parents, and sometimes by the child himself or herself. This year they were found on your child's head.

Lice are very common wherever groups of people congregate. Schools, orphanages, military establishments, and other institutions must constantly be on the alert because if the condition is not discovered early, it spreads from person to person very rapidly. It can spread by direct scalp-to-scalp contact or by children using the same comb, cap, or scarf or by sleeping in the same bed.

The head louse is a small, thin, greyish insect about 1/4 inch long and is found in the scalp. It lives by biting the skin of the scalp and eating the blood that comes through the bite. Children with lice often get sores and boils on their head because the bits get infected very easily. Lice lay their eggs directly on the hair, close to the scalp. These eggs are called "nits" and are actually stuck to the hair. Scales of dandruff can be found on the hair or scalp, but they are always loose and not stuck on to the hair. The eggs or "nits" hatch out into adult lice in 8 to 10 days.

It is not difficult to treat lice, but it does take time and persistence. The medicine will kill the adult lice, but nothing kills the eggs or "nits." There are many medicines that may be used. You should consult your family physician or the school nurse for advice as to the proper treatment.

The district is authorized to exclude children from school who have pediculosis (lice). The child will not be admitted in school until inspection or doctor's statement reveals that the infestation has cleared up.

_____

School

PEDICULOSIS INFORMATION LETTER
(Spanish)

Estimado padre de familia:

Durante cada año escolar a muchos de los niños se les ha encontrado tener piojos. Algunas veces son descubiertos por la maestra, otras veces por los papas y en ocasiónes por el niño mismo. Este año fueron encontrados en el cabello de su niño.

Los piojos son muy comunes en cualquier lugar donde se juntan grupos de gente. Escuelas, orfanatorios, establecimientos militares y otras instituciones deben estar constantemente en alerta debido a que si la condición no es descubierta a tiempo, se extiende de persona a persona muy rápidamente. Se puede extender del contacto directo de cráneo á cráneo o por niños que usen el mismo peine, por el uso de gorras o pañoletas ajenas o por dormir en la misma cama.

El piojo principal es un insecto grisaceo y pequeño de aproximadamente 1/4 de pulgada de largo y se halla en el cráneo. Se alimenta picando la piel del cráneo y comiendose la sangre que resulta de ella. Niños con piojos suelen adquirir granos en la cabeza ya que los piquetes se infectan muy fácilmente. Los piojos ponen sus huevos directamente en el cabello cerca del cráneo. Estos huevos se llaman liendres y efectivamente se pegan al cabello. La caspa se puede encontrar en el cabello o en el cráneo pero siempre está suelta y no pegada al cabello. Los huevos o las liendres se convierten en piojos en ocho o diez dias.

No es difícil el tratamiento para eliminar los piojos, pero si se requiere tiempo y persistencia. La medicina mata los piojos pero no mata los huevos o las liendres. Por consiguiente recomendamos el tratamiento el primer día, el quinto día y el décimo día y así hasta matar todos los piojos que se desarrollen en el curso de los diez días.

Este distrito está autorizado de excluir de la escuela a niños que tienen piojos. El niño(a) no sera admitido(a) en la escuela hasta que inspección o declaración de un doctor sea recibida manifestando que la condición se ha terminado.

_____
Escolar

TREATMENT OF NITS WITH VINEGAR
(English)

Nits, or eggs, will stay on the hair after the lice are killed. To remove the nits, the following treatment is recommended that will soften the material that holds the nits to the hair. If the nits, or eggs, are not combed out or removed, they will hatch and become lice.

1. Mix 1 quart vinegar and 1 quart water.
2. Wet large towel with water and vinegar.
3. Wring out the towel and wrap it around the person's head.
4. Leave the towel on the head for 2 hours.
5. Remove towel and comb the hair with a fine-toothed comb to remove nits.
6. Shampoo and rinse hair well.
7. Repeat treatment as needed.

TRATAMIENTO PARA LIENDRES USANDO VINAGRE
(Spanish)

Las liendres se quedan en el cabello después que se mueren los piojos. Para quitar las liendres, el tratamiento que sigue es recomendado. Para removerlas, es necesario suavizar el material que hace que las liendres se peguen al cabello. Si las liendres no se quitan, nacerán de nuevo y se haran piojos.

1. Mezcle 1 cuarto de vinagre y l cuarto de agua. Esta solución se puede calentar un poco a que este tibia.
2. Moje una toalla grande con el agua y el vinagre.
3. Exprima la toalla y envuélvale la cabeza a la persona en la toalla.
4. Deje la toalla en la cabeza por dos horas.
5. Quite la toalla y peine el cabello con un peine de dientes tupidos.
6. Lave y enjuague bien el cabello.
7. Repita el tratamiento cuando sea necesario.

INSTRUCTIONS FOR THE USE OF KWELL LOTION
(English)

Apply to dry hair the amount necessary to wet the hair but never more than 2 ounces. Leave the lotion on the hair. Rinse hair well at the end of the time period instructed.

If lice are still living after seven days, repeat treatment *one* more time only. Do not use Kwell more than a total of two times within a thirty-day period. Use only as recommended. To be used for students enrolled in the school district.

INSTRUCCIONES PARA EL USO DE LOCION KWELL
(Spanish)

Aplique al cabello seco la cantidad necesaria para mojar el cabello pero no más de 2 onzas. Al fin de las horas instruidas lave y enjuague bien el cabello. Si después de 7 días todavía hay piojos vivos, repita el tratamiento solamente *una* vez más. No use la loción Kwell mas de 2 veces durante un periodo de 30 dias. Use solo como se recomienda. La loción debe ser usada solamente por los estudiantes matriculados en el distrito escolar.

NURSE'S REPORT OF COMMUNICABLE DISEASE

_____   _____
School   Date

_____   _____   _____   _____
Pupil   Address   Telephone   Age

Grade K 1 2 3 4 5 6 7 8 9 10 11 12; Sex M F   **Race:**

☐ American Indian or Alaskan Native
☐ Asian or Pacific Islander
☐ Black, not of Hispanic origin
☐ Hispanic
☐ White, not of Hispanic origin

Diseases reported by name, age, sex, race, and diagnosing physician

☐ Diphtheria   ☐ Measles (rubella)   ☐ Pertussis
☐ Hepatitis, infectious ☐ Meningitis, aseptic   ☐ Poliomyelitis
☐ Hepatitis, serum   ☐ Meningitis, bacterial ☐ Venereal disease
☐ Measles (rubeola)   ☐ Mumps   ☐ Other

Diseases Reported by Number Only:

Pediculosis _____

Family Members Rx'd _____

Scabies _____

Ringworm of Scalp _____

Date kept from school by parent or guardian _____

Date readmitted to class _____ Days absent _____

Doctor _____ Teacher _____

Doctor's phone _____

COMMUNICABLE DISEASE CHART

Disease	Incubation period	Early signs of illness	Isolation	Notes
Athlete's foot	Unknown.	Blisters and cracking of the skin of the feet, usually between the toes.	Not excluded from school. Suspected cases should be excluded from gymnasiums, swimming pools, and activities likely to lead to exposure of others.	Teach importance of hygienic care. Refer to private physician or Health Department.
Chickenpox	2 to 3 weeks.	Slight fever, fine blisters appear first on scalp, then on face and body. Successive crops of blisters remain 3 to 4 days, leaving scabs.	Six days after last crop of blisters appear.	No vaccine available. Consult your physician.
Common cold	12 to 72 hours. Usually 24 hours.	Runny nose, watery eyes, chilliness and malaise. Usually no fever, unless complications have developed.	Until clinical recovery.	
Diphtheria	2 to 5 days, occasionally longer.	Sore throat, fever, the symptoms rapidly become more severe.	Until two cultures from both nose and throat, taken after cessation of antimicrobial therapy and not less than 24 hours apart, fail to yield diphtheria bacilli.	Vaccine available. Consult your physician or Health Department.
Epidemic meningitis	Varies from 2 to 10 days. Commonly 3 to 4 days.	Sudden onset of headache, fever, nausea and often vomiting, stiff neck. Frequently a fine spotted rash appears.	Exclude from school until released by private physician or Health Department.	Consult your physician.
Head lice (pediculosis)	Eggs hatch in a week; reach sexual maturity in about 2 weeks.	Excessive scratching of head. White egg (nit) on hair that will not flick off.	Exclude until under treatment.	Refer to private physician or Health Department.
Viral hepatitis A. Infectious	From 15 to 50 days. Usually 25 days.	Nausea, vomiting, extreme fatigue, often pain in upper abdomen followed by jaundice. Mild cases occur without jaundice in children.	Exclude from school until released by private physician or Health Department.	Supervised handwashing after using the toilet and before meals will help control spread. Personal hygiene is emphasized. See your physician.
B. Serum	45 to 160 days. Average 60 to 90 days.	Masked onset, loss of appetite, vague abdominal discomfort, nausea, vomiting, often progressing to jaundice	Exclude from school until released from medical supervision.	
Impetigo	Variable.	Small blisters on the skin which later become crusted and contain pus.	Permit school attendance if under adequate treatment.	Refer to private physician or Health Department.
Influenza	24 to 72 hours.	Rapid onset with fever, chills, headache, lack of energy, muscle aching, sore throat, cough	Until clinical recovery.	
Measles—Rubeola	7 to 14 days.	Runny nose, watery eyes, fever, cough. Blotchy rash appears fourth day.	During catarrhal state and for 7 days after appearance of rash.	Vaccine available. Consult your physician or Health Department.
German Measles—Rubella	14 to 21 days.	Slight head cold. Swollen, tender glands at back of neck. Changeable rash.	Until clinical recovery.	Vaccine available. Consult your physician or Health Department.
Mumps	12 to 26 days.	Pain in cheeks, increased by chewing. Swelling over the jaw and in front of ear.	Until swelling disappears.	Vaccine available. See your physician.
Pink eye—conjunctivitis	Usually 24 to 72 hours.	Red eyes, discharge from eyes, crusted lids.	Exclude until released by private physician.	Consult your physician.
Poliomyelitis	Commonly 7 to 12 days with a range from 3 to 21 days.	Fever, headache, malaise, gastrointestinal disturbance, stiffness of the neck and back. Often followed by paralysis.	Exclude from school until released by physician or Health Department.	Can be prevented by vaccination. See your physician or Health Department.

Disease	Incubation period	Early signs of illness	Isolation	Notes
Rickettsial Disease A. Rocky Mountain Spotted Fever	3 to 10 days.	Sudden onset, moderate to high fever, ordinarily persisting 2 to 3 weeks, headaches, chills, redness of eyes. Raised rash on extremities progressing to palms and soles	Not necessary.	Transmitted by tick bites. Not directly communicable from person to person.
B. Typhus	1 to 2 weeks.	Headaches, chills, lack of energy, fever, aches, raised rash appearing on the fifth or sixth day.	Not necessary.	Transmitted by flea bites. Not directly communicable from person to person.
Ringworm of the body	4 to 10 days.	Flat, spreading, scaly, ring-shaped spots. The margins are usually reddish and elevated.	Permit school attendance if under adequate treatment and sores are covered.	Refer to private physician or Health Department.
Ringworm of the scalp	10 to 14 days.	Flat spreading, ring-shaped bald spots on hairy parts of head.	Exclude unless under adequate treatment. Consult Health Department for current regulations.	Refer to private physician or Health Department.
Salmonellosis	6 to 72 hours.	Sudden onset, abdominal pain, diarrhea, nausea, vomiting and fever.	Exclude until released by physician.	
Scabies	Several days or weeks.	Small raised reddened areas or blisters with connecting grayish-white lines. Marked itching. Most commonly found in folds of the skin.	Exclude until under adequate treatment and no open lesions can be observed.	Refer to private physician or Health Department.
Shigellosis	1 to 7 days.	Diarrhea, cramps, fever, vomiting.	Exclude from school until released by physician.	
Streptococcal infections (including scarlet fever)	1 to 3 days.	Fever, sore throat. Fine red rash over body for scarlet fever.	For at least 7 days from onset if untreated. With adequate medical treatment, 48 hours.	No vaccine available. Consult your physician.
Tetanus	4 days to 3 weeks	Painful muscular contractions primarily of the masseter (jaw) and neck muscles.	Not necessary.	Vaccine available. Consult physician or Health Department.
Tuberculosis	4 to 12 weeks from infection to demonstrable pulmonary lesion.	Listlessness, loss of appetite, weight loss, low-grade fever, positive tuberculin skin test.	Case: If proved to be noninfectious and physical condition permits, may attend school. Contacts: May attend school but should have TB skin tests. If positive, child should be referred to his family physician for further study.	If reactor prevalence is 1% or greater, recommend TB skin tests of first and seventh grade school children to identify tuberculin reactors for referral to physician for further study.
Venereal disease A. Gonorrhea	3 to 5 days	Male: Purulent urethral discharge; burning on urination; inflammation and swelling of genital region. Female: Possibly no symptoms; vaginal discharge, pain in abdomen (when salpingitis occurs).	Not necessary	Refer to private physician or Health Department. National Venereal Disease Hotline—1-800-227-8922—toll free.
B. Syphilis	21 days	First sign: genital sore (5-week duration); Second sign: generalized rash, mucous patches, sore throat, headache, fever alopecia, etc. (7-week duration).	Not necessary	Refer to private physician or Health Department. National Venereal Disease Hotline—1-800-227-8922—toll free.
Whooping cough Pertussis	7 to 10 days	Tight dry cough that becomes more severe. Cough, whoop, and vomit.	For 21 days after appearance of typical "whoop."	Vaccine available. Consult your physician or Health Department.

FORMS FOR
THE DENTAL PROGRAM

DENTAL RECORD OF FILLINGS AND EXTRACTIONS

The records are used to keep a permanent record of all dental therapy (fillings, extractions, and so on) done at a school that uses dentists, dental hygienists, or trained dental assistants.

Many school districts offer dental health education to their students; not many offer actual dental therapy. For those that do, standard dental records are helpful.

DENTAL PERMIT

School _____

Dear Parent:

     Through the teeth care program your child is eligible for dental care. The dental work will be done by a dentist in a mobile clinic located at the school. There is no charge. This work may include cleaning, fluoridation, X rays, extractions, and fillings depending on what the dentist feels is necessary.

     I give my permission for my child _____ _____to

                                         Name   Date of birth

receive dental work as described above.

Please check

1. **My child has allergies:**   Yes _____   No _____   If so, what _____

2. **My child is on medication:**   Yes _____   No _____   If so, what _____

3. **My child has a long-term illness:** Yes _____   No _____   If so, what _____

_____   _____
    Parent or guardian signature   **Date**

_____   _____
          Address   **Phone**

REPORT OF SCHOOL DENTAL INSPECTION

Student's name _____ **Grade** _____ **Teacher** _____

Dear Parent or Guardian:

A school dental inspection has been made. The inspection gives a *general* idea as to the condition of your child's teeth but *does not* take the place of a thorough examination in your dentist's office.

As a result of this inspection, we wish to

_____ Commend you for the dental care that has been provided and urge that it be continued.

_____ Inform you of the need for dental attention.

_____ Urge immediate dental attention. Ill health, pain, and increasing expense can be avoided by prompt dental treatment.

Please check one of the following statements and return the lower part of this sheet to school.

Thank you,

_____
School nurse

_____

Detach here and return

Student's name _____ **Grade** _____ **Teacher** _____

_____ My child receives regular dental care and was last seen by the dentist on _____ (date).

_____ I have made an appointment with a dentist to have the necessary work done.

_____ I will make an appointment to have the needed work done.

_____ I am unable to make the needed appointment.

Comments _____

_____

_____

_____
Parent's or guardian's signature

INSTRUCTIONS AFTER TOOTH REMOVAL

1. The child is kept in the dental van until bleeding has stopped; however, on return to class, there may be some "oozing" and the saliva may be pink.

2. The child may eat lunch and should be encouraged to do so.

3. The child may drink water but *should not* rinse his or her mouth by swishing the water and spitting.

4. The parent may give the child aspirin for pain, but it should be swallowed, *not* held next to the sore spot.

FORMS FOR EVALUATION AND OBSERVATION OF SCHOOL NURSES AND AIDES

The type of form chosen by a school district reflects the detail and objectivity desired by that district in its evaluation. Some forms are subjective, some are more detailed. A variety are included here to reflect the purpose needed.

STAFF ORIENTATION CHECKLIST

This checklist will be useful in planning a new staff person's orientation schedule.

Subject	Date discussed	By whom
1. Organizational structure		
2. Role of coordinator		
3. Role of central office staff		
4. Role of nurse practitioner		
5. Role of health aide I		
6. Role of health aide II (LVN)		
7. Role of R.N. supervisor		
8. Policies and procedures		
9. Reporting absenteeism		
10. _____ Nursing association		
11. Flow of communication by: • In-house courier system • Telephone calling committee • Other		
12. R.N., LVN, HA schedules		
13. Performance review process		
14. Dress code (I.D. tag)		
15. Annual report of immunization status		
16. Items to be returned upon termination of employment		
17. Coordination of special activities: T.B. testing, physicals, etc.		
18. Active immunization procedures manual		
19. *Handbook of Administrative Procedures and Programs* a. Administrative procedures b. School health programs c. Medical protocols and standing orders d. Communicable/infectious diseases e. Forms f. Information letters		
20. School health program chart (local/federal)		

SCHOOL NURSE EVALUATION
(Confidential)

Employee's name

_____

Last   **First**   **Middle**

Recommendation of Principal

☐ **Recommended for reemployment**

☐ **Not recommended for reemployment**

Nurse's Statement

A formal conference was held on (date) _____ **with my principal.**

I acknowledge that each of the personal and professional characteristics listed within was discussed and that specific suggestions were recommended. I understand that my signature below does not necessarily mean that I agree with the evaluation. I also understand that I have the right to discuss my status with the school superintendent.

Signed comments are attached by principal ☐ **and/or nurse** ☐

Date _____   **Nurse's signature** _____

School _____   **Nurse's social security number** _____

                                             Principal's signature _____

Nurse's Overall Rating

                     Successful   **Marginal**   **Unsuccessful**
                          ☐   ☐   ☐

Nursing assignment _____

Number of years of service, including this year, in this school _____

Current years of service, including this year, in the school district _____

Total years of service in community health nursing _____

Comments _____

_____

_____

_____

_____

_____

SCHOOL NURSE EVALUATION
Page 2

Nurse _____ **Nurse** assignment _____ Date _____

I. Personal-Professional Preparedness

Successful   Marginal   Unsuccessful
□   □   □

Comments

A. Fulfills professional role expectations with minimal personal–family interest conflict.

B. Reflects professional leadership abilities in mature self-directed goal-setting, decision-making, and action-taking activities.

C. Demonstrates capacity to alter self-rewarding attitudes and behavior in interest of providing assistance to pupils, peers, and community.

D. Supports philosophy of school health services program by maintaining a life-style that reduces tardiness and absenteeism to a minimum.

E. Participates in self-directed, ongoing learning activities for acquisition of new knowledge and skills for upgrading school nurse practice.

II. Health Room Management

Successful   Marginal   Unsuccessful
□   □   □

Comments

A. Creates emotional and physical environment conducive to the maintenance of safe, orderly, and attractive work area.

B. Develops full functioning health program through maximum utilization of existing facility.

C. Anticipates supply and equipment needs appropriate for maintaining a continuous, functional school health program.

D. Develops a program that assures safe ongoing emergency health care in the absence of the nurse.

E. Initiates planning for appropriate communication with principal and faculty to ensure ongoing health program with minimal interruption to total building schedule.

F. Maintains accurate, updated records of health information on all students and makes provision for the timely and accurate management of incoming and outgoing records and reports.

G. Initiates referrals and follow-up relevant to unmet health needs of students and makes appropriate distribution of health information to facilitate recommended change in academic schedule.

III. Pupil-Nurse Relationships

Successful   Marginal   Unsuccessful
□   □   □

Comments

A. Demonstrates an honest, caring attitude that invites student trust.

Nurse _____ Nurse assignment _____ Date _____

III. Pupil-Nurse Relationships (continued)

Comments

B. Demonstrates a capacity to see student as a total person rather than a physical, social, or educational problem. _____

C. Demonstrates consistent behavior in assisting students with management of health problems. _____

D. Possesses resourcefulness and skill in assisting students with health maintenance needs. _____

E. Respects human need to treat personal health problems as a very private affair. _____

IV. Practice Skills and Knowledge

A. Health Service

Successful ☐   Marginal ☐   Unsuccessful ☐

Comments

1. Practices within the defined limits of school district policy. _____

2. Possesses skills appropriate for meeting school health emergencies. _____

3. Demonstrates full range of knowledge and skills in health appraisal techniques. _____

4. Coordinates total health program with related building-level activities and serves as health team leader to participating personnel. _____

5. Allocates appropriate job function to support personnel. _____

6. Utilizes appropriate resources within the school and community to promote optimum delivery of health care services. _____

7. Anticipates building-level health maintenance needs and serves as health team leader in school-community activities for communicable disease control, preschool health screening, health room volunteer services, etc. _____

B. Health Counseling

Successful ☐   Marginal ☐   Unsuccessful ☐

Comments

1. Demonstrates a sensitivity to students' need to be heard as well as to be helped. _____

2. Interprets and utilizes health information with good judgment and professional skill. _____

3. Demonstrates understanding and mastery of role function for constructive participation in pupil-personnel activities. _____

4. Serves as a role model in professional management of student and family confidences in team interaction situations. _____

5. Assists students, parents, and school faculty in exploring alternate approaches to meeting health care needs. _____

6. Participates in a helping relationship with individuals or families in crisis intervention. _____

7. Initiates planning for teacher-nurse conferences at appropriate intervals to consider the physical, social, and emotional health of each child. _____

Nurse _____ Nurse assignment _____ Date _____

C. Health Education

Successful	Marginal	Unsuccessful
☐	☐	☐

Comments

1. Utilizes health service activities as a vehicle for direct and indirect health teaching. _____
2. Makes accurate assessments of health education needs pertinent to school, community and the individual. _____
3. Serves as resource person to school faculty and nurse staff in special areas of expertise. _____
4. Recognizes self-limitations in speciality areas and compensates deficiencies by involving appropriate resource persons from the health-medical community in the educational process. _____
5. Provides creative learning experiences relevant to health information needs to equip students to make constructive decisions regarding health behavior. _____
6. Possesses knowledge and skill for creative adaptation of accurate and timely health concepts to the educational process. _____
7. Services as an extension to career education efforts through knowledgeable and creative participation in area of health career guidance. _____

V. Public Relations

Successful	Marginal	Unsuccessful
☐	☐	☐

Comments

1. Assists in establishing and maintaining a positive school-community relationship. _____
2. Demonstrates a capacity for responding to the many publics in a positive and constructive manner. _____
3. Participates in active role with appropriate health and welfare representatives of PTA. _____
4. Interprets and conducts school health program in a manner that elicits positive supports from students, parents, school, and community. _____
5. Communicates, through creative participation, a vital interest in community health. _____
6. Recognizes the parent to be an extension of the school health program and invites parent involvement in health care planning. _____

VI. Health and Appearance

Successful	Marginal	Unsuccessful
☐	☐	☐

Comments

1. Keeps grooming and personal attire appropriate to professional duties of school nurse practice. _____
2. Contributes to the positive image of school health programs through the practice of good health habits. _____
3. Maintains poise and stability in students, parent, and peer group relationship. _____
4. Demonstrates vigor and vitality in the performance of duties. _____

SCHOOL NURSING EVALUATION FORMS FOR ADMINISTRATORS AND SCHOOL NURSE SUPERVISORS

I. Responsibility to the school staff

1. Demonstrates professional nursing ability and knowledge of developmental, clinical, and educational processes. _____
2. Has interpreted and alerted the school administrator to school health laws, problems, and trends. _____
3. Has established effective relations with school personnel and community patrons. _____

II. Health appraisal

1. Has conducted all required health assessment screening programs. _____
2. Uses information gathered from health assessment techniques to identify health problems. _____
3. Makes valid referrals to pupils, parents, and teachers for remediation recommendation and educational program adaptation for identifiable health problems. _____
4. Uses a system of periodic review and supervision of all pupils' health status. _____

III. Health counseling

1. Has identified pupils in need of health counseling. _____
2. Has effectively conducted individual and group health counseling sessions with pupils and parents. _____
3. Makes valid referrals to appropriate school and community resources. _____

IV. Special education programs

1. Serves effectively on admission and dismissal committees. _____
2. Continuously keeps special teachers informed of pupils' health status. _____

SCHOOL NURSE EVALUATION FORM

*O Outstanding   Performance as observed is consistently exceptional and is worthy of special recognition.

C Competent   Performance as observed is professionally competent and meets expectations of district.

N Needs improvement   Performance as observed indicates a need for continued growth, and improvement is expected.

*U Unacceptable   Performance as observed does not meet the standards of district and improvement is mandatory.

*Comments must be recorded

Performance competencies	O	C	N	U	Comments
1.00 Personal-professional characteristics					
1.01 Fulfills professional role expectations with minimal personal interest–family conflict.					
1.02 Reflects professional leadership abilities in responsible self-directed goal-setting, decision-making, and action-taking activities.					
1.03 Exercises professional judgment in absences from work.					
1.04 Participates in self-directed continuing learning activities in acquiring new skills and knowledge for upgrading school nursing.					
2.00 Health clinic management					
2.01 Maintains a safe, orderly, and attractive work area with appropriate emotional and physical environment.					
2.02 Develops a program that assures safe ongoing emergency health care.					
2.03 Anticipates supply and equipment needs for maintaining and continuous school health program.					
2.04 Develops a complete and functioning health program through maximum utilization of existing facilities.					
2.05 Plans for communication with principals and faculties to provide a health program with minimal interruption to total building schedule.					
2.06 Maintains accurate and current health information on all students to ensure the timely management of incoming and outgoing records and reports.					
2.07 Initiates referrals and follow-up relevant to the unmet health needs.					
2.08 Makes appropriate distribution of health information to facilitate recommended changes in academic schedules.					
3.00 Interacting with students					
3.01 Provides opportunities for developing self-evaluation skills that aid the student in setting realistic goals and understanding himself, his strengths, and his limitations.					
3.02 Assists the student in accepting responsibility for his or her actions.					

Performance competencies	O	C	N	U	Comments
3.03 Demonstrates respect for students by showing tolerance for students whose ideas differ; using supportive criticism rather than blame, shame, or sarcasm; encouraging students to respect the rights of others; being fair, impartial, and objective in the treatment of students.					
3.04 Provides opportunities for all students to experience success by recognizing the special needs of students.					
3.05 Utilizes appropriate district services available to benefit the student.					
3.06 Sets an example of, and encourages, socially acceptable behavior.					
3.07 Maintains an atmosphere conducive to freedom of thought and expression and shows respect for pupil opinions and suggestions.					
3.08 Readily available to students for counseling and individual help.					
4.00 Professional attitude and conduct					
4.01 Shows an honest, caring attitude that invites student trust.					
4.02 Demonstrates the ability to see student as a total person rather than a physical, educational or social problem.					
4.03 Uses resourcefulness and skill in helping students with health maintenance needs and with management of health problems.					
4.04 Respects the need to treat personal health problems as a very private affair.					
5.00 Skills and knowledge					
5.01 Demonstrates knowledge and skills in health appraisal techniques.					
5.02 Utilizes appropriate resources within the community to promote delivery of health care services.					
5.03 Serves as a leader in school community activities for communicable disease control, preschool health screening, health room volunteer services, etc.					
5.04 Demonstrates a sensitivity to student's need to be heard as well as helped by health counseling.					
5.05 Interprets and uses health information with good judgment					
5.06 Helps students and parents in exploring alternate approaches to meeting health care needs.					
5.07 Provides a helping relationship with individuals or families in crises intervention.					
5.08 Participates in teacher-nurse-family conferences at appropriate times to consider the physical, emotional, and social health of each child.					
6.00 Health education skills					
6.01 Uses health services activities as a vehicle for direct and indirect health teaching.					
6.02 Serves as a resource person to the school staff in special areas of expertise.					
6.03 Involves appropriate resource persons from the health-medical community in the educational process.					
6.04 Provide learning experiences to equip students to make constructive decisions regarding health behavior.					
6.05 Serves as an extension to career education efforts through participation in the area of health career guidance.					

Performance competencies	O	C	N	U	Comments
7.00 Interacting with parents and community					
7.01 Contributes to establishing and maintaining a positive school-community relationship.					
7.02 Participates in an active role with health, welfare, and community activities.					
7.03 Conducts the school health program in a manner that elicits positive support from students, parents, school, and community.					
7.04 Communicates an interest in community health through creative participation.					
7.05 Recognizes that the parent is an extension of the school health program and invites parental involvement in planning health care.					
8.00 Appearance and health					
8.01 Keeps grooming and personal attire appropriate to professional health services practice.					
8.02 Increases the positive image of school health programs through the practice of good health habits.					
8.03 Maintains stability and poise in student, parent, and peer group relationships.					
8.04 Demonstrates enthusiasm and vitality in the performance of duties.					

NEW LVN EVALUATION FORM

Rating scale:				Date																	Comments
Exceeds expectations	(3)																					
Meets expectations	(2)																					
Needs improvement	(1)																					
Unable to observe	(0)	Campus																				

I. *Clinic practices:* For each item consider knowledge, planning, execution, recording, and notification of parent or school personnel.
- A. Minor first aid
- B. Advanced first aid
- C. Acute health problems
- D. Chronic health problems

II. *Clinic management:* Consider knowledge and practice.
- A. Supplies—adequate stock, ordering
- B. Cleanliness and order
- C. Safety

III. *Immunization program:* Consider knowledge, practice, and use of resources.
- A. Determining student's immunization status
- B. Use of CD permits
- C. Administration of vaccines
- D. Recording
- E. Parental notification

Rating scale:

   Exceeds expectations   (3)   **Date**

   Meets expectations   (2)

   Needs improvement   (1)

   Unable to observe   (0)   **Campus**   **Comments**

IV. *Medication program:* Consider knowledge and practice.

   A. Obtaining parental and physician permission.

   B. Dispensing practices

   C. Recording

   D. Reporting as required

   E. Use of emergency insect sting kit

V. *Student services:* For each item, consider knowledge, planning, execution, recording, notification of parent or school personnel, use of resources, referral, and follow-up.

   A. Screening physical assessments

   B. Tuberculosis testing

   C. Special education referral and appraisal process

   D. Special Olympics (health portion)

   E. Nutrition education

   F. Dental health education

   G. Health education

   H. Dental program

      1. Chapter I regular

      2. Chapter 2 migrant

Rating scale:																		Comments
Exceeds expectations (3) **Date**																		
Meets expectations (2)																		
Needs improvement (1)																		
Unable to observe (0) **Campus**																		

VI. *Screening tests:* Consider knowledge, planning, execution, technique, recording, notification of parents and school personnel, use of resources, referral, and follow-up.
  - A. Vision screening
    1. Acuity
    2. Latent hyperopia
  - B. Hearing screening
  - C. Growth assessment
  - D. Dental screening
  - E. B/P screening
  - F. Hematocrit
  - G. Urinalysis

VII. *Procedural and record-keeping skills:* Consider compliance with policy, accuracy, and neatness.
  - A. Clinic log (basic)
  - B. Clinic log (chapter I)
  - C. Health records
  - D. Permanent cumulative records
  - E. Monthly reports
  - F. Annual reports
  - G. Chapter I regular program
  - H. Home visits
  - I. Parent conference

Rating scale:

Exceeds expectations (3) **Date**														
Meets expectations (2)														
Needs improvement (1)														
Unable to observe (0) **Campus**													**Comments**

VIII. Personal and professional qualities

   A. Assumes responsibility for own professional growth.

   B. Fosters positive self-image in students.

   C. Cooperates with co-workers and supervisors.

   D. Plans and prioritizes work

   E. Demonstrates initiative

   F. Demonstrates adaptability

   G. Has positive relationship with students, staff, and parents.

   H. Complies with dress code

Comments: (Use space to describe personal characteristics or special activities not addressed above.)

_____

_____

_____	_____	_____	_____
Nursing supervisor	R.N. coordinator	LVN	Date

EXPERIENCED LVN EVALUATION FORM

Name	Date	School assignment

Rating scale: Exceed expectations   (3)*
Meets expectations   (2)
Needs improvement   (1)*
Unable to observe   (0)

Performance competencies	3	2	1	0	Comments
A. Personal-professional characteristics					
1. Exhibits appropriate response to job-related situations.					
2. Demonstrates initiative.					
3. Communicates effectively with students, staff and parents.					
4. Observes the policies and procedures of the school district and department.					
5. Is prompt and accurate in handling records, reports, and materials.					
6. Develops and utilizes well-organized plans for the year.					
7. Is reliable and conscientious in adhering to the school's time schedule.					
8. Complies with dress code.					
9. Cooperates with co-workers and supervisors.					
10. Assumes responsibility for own professional growth.					
B. Health clinic management					
1. Maintains a safe and attractive clinic.					
2. Plans and orders clinic supplies in advance of need.					
3. Maintains up-to-date reports and records and keeps information confidential.					
C. Skills and knowledge					
1. Demonstrates knowledge and skills in health appraisal techniques.					
2. Makes appropriate referrals and pursues follow-up to referrals.					
3. Knows and utilizes community resources.					
4. Interprets and uses health information with good judgment.					
5. Handles first aid and emergency care calmly and efficiently.					
6. Informs teachers of student's medical problems and proper procedure for handling them.					
7. Fosters positive self-image in students.					
8. Uses health services activities as a vehicle for direct and indirect health teaching.					

Nurse coordinator's signature _____ Date _____

LVN's signature† _____ Date _____

*Comments must be recorded.
†Signature does not necessarily imply agreement. It indicates that the person has seen the evaluation. If there is disagreement, LVN may comment in space below.

SUPERVISOR'S EVALUATION OF HEALTH AIDE

Rating scale
  S Satisfactory
  U Unsatisfactory

I. First Aid Practices
  A. Minor Problems
  B. Handling of major problems

II. Clinic Management
  A. Supplies
  B. Cleanliness
  C. Safety

III. Medication
  A. Dispensing practices
  B. Recording
  C. Keeps R.N. informed

IV. Height and weight
  A. Completes assignment
  B. Recording
  C. Use of height/weight charts

V. Nutrition education
  A. Preparation of assignment
  B. Completion of assignment

VI. Visions (acuity and hyperopia)
  A. Completes assignment
  B. Recording

VII. Dental
  A. Screening
  B. Education

Date
Campus

Rating

	Date
	Campus

VIII. Urine Screening
  A. Performance
  B. Interpretation of results

IX. Other screening procedures (assisting with)
  A. Performance

X. Use of thermometer
  A. Clean technique
  B. Accurate reading
  C. Reporting of elevated temperature

XI. Policies
  A. Follows instructions

XII. Use of time
  A. Punctual
  B. Organizes work schedule

XIII. Record keeping
  A. Clinic log (Basic)
  B. Clinic log (Title I)
  C. Medication record
  D. Health record
  E. Monthly reports

XIV. Dress Code

XV. Personal Relationships
  A. Students
  B. Staff
  C. Parents

Comments:

_____

H/A signature

_____

Date

FORMS FOR HEALTH FILE FOR EACH STUDENT

CUMULATIVE HEALTH RECORDS

The cumulative health record, often simply called the "health card," is probably the most widely used form in most school districts and exists in many formats. Of the examples shown here, some are relatively simple, whereas others are more complex and inclusive.

This health record is meant to accompany the child throughout his or her school career. A major problem is lost records; therefore, it is important that the format of the health card physically fits into (or onto) the student's academic and attendance permanent record card. Many health cards are lost when students move from elementary to middle or junior high school and again moving from middle to high school. If the health card is constructed to match and be compatible with the academic record form, fewer health cards will be lost.

When the student graduates from high school, the health record becomes part of the total permanent record. Immunizations as well as records of chronic illnesses are available for college entrance, military service, and future employment. Because certain stigmatizing chronic illness, such as epilepsy, are sometimes erased from the health card when the student graduates (a practice that may be criticized as tampering with records), a sheet called Nurse's Notes can be used and discarded when the student graduates. The nurse's notes can simply be viewed as a working sheet to record events that help in the child's health management. In the view of some authorities, these working sheets need not be surrendered. The school district's attorney should be consulted. In the absence of a nurse, the form can be labeled Health Notes.

The K-12 student health record serves as a supplement to the student's scholastic cumulative record. Health record entries are made only by the nurse/nurse aide staff and attention should be given to the quality and authority of all health data entries.

All recordings done should be in permanent black ink only. Recording the results of health appraisals is done in the column under the grade designated. For example, for children in kindergarten, data will be recorded in the column designated K. Data for students in third grade will be recorded in column 3, and so on.

For state auditing purposes, close attention should be given to the accuracy of all immunization data entries, including date of dosages of a series and name of verifying physician or health agency.

This health record is transferred from school to school with the cumulative record when the student remains in the particular school district. If the student moves out of the school district, the record should be filed in a "Dropped" file in the last school the student attended. Records to be destroyed should be put in a box or envelope and given to the custodian to be incinerated.

Cumulative health records of regular education students should be kept in the school clinic file until the student's twenty-first birthday. Health records of students who attended special education classes should be kept in the school clinic file until a student's twenty-third birthday. Relevant health information on special education students is in each student's special education file and should be handled separately in the way that department so chooses.

NURSE'S NOTES

The purpose of the Nurse's Notes (or Health Notes) is to record health notes other than mandated items (such as immunizations, vision, hearing, or scoliosis exams) to augment the permanent record card.

For example,

1. *Diagnoses of long-term illness or disability:* An educational diagnosis of emotional disability, learning disability, or dyslexia; a medical diagnosis of epilepsy or attention-deficit disorder; or conduct disorder may adversely effect a child's future if recorded on the permanent record card, even though such symptoms may be completely outgrown by high school graduation.

2. *Changes of medication for chronic illness:* This requires more space than is available on the health card. To obtain the needed space, some nurses enter the medication dose in pencil, erase when the dose is changed and write in a new dose. Using this form, the total record of medication dosage is not lost.

3. *Reports of all forms of child abuse:* Space is required to report follow-up and disposition of each case.

If the Nurses Notes sheet is to be folded in half and filed with the health card, it should be slightly smaller so it will not protrude from the edges of the health card and get in the way when it is necessary to search through the health cards.

CUMULATIVE RECORD—HEALTH INSERT

LAST NAME   FIRST NAME   MIDDLE NAME

Rev 8/83 with the cooperation of the California School Nurses Organization

CUMULATIVE RECORD—HEALTH INSERT
Confidential Information for use by Professional Personnel   FORM HL—K P Graphics, Roseville CA • 1983

BIRTHDATE — Month / Day / Year   Check Sex   M ☐   F ☐

	YEAR
GRADE	
TEACHER	

IMMUNIZATION & TEST RECORD
Enter Month and Year   EXEMPT Medical Reasons

POLIO	
DPT/Td	
MEASLES (10 day)	
RUBELLA (3 day)	
MUMPS	
TUBERCULIN	
OTHER	

Please check below if any problems are present:

Known Eye Problems:
☐ Glasses ☐ Contact Lens ☐ Preferential Seating
Under care of Dr. ____

Known Hearing Problems:
☐ Hearing Aid ☐ Preferential Seating
Under care of Dr. ____

P = passed   F = failed   5   6   7   8

SCOLIOSIS: Screening [ ]   Rescreening [ ]   Referred Date, ____   Referred Date ____

SIGNIFICANT HEALTH HISTORY

	YEAR		YEAR
Asthma		Hepatitis	
Birth Defect		Mono	
Bone, Joint or Muscle Problems		Mumps	
Chickenpox		Rheumatic Fever	
Diabetes		Scarlet Fever	
Excessive Colds		Seizure Disorder	
Frequent Ear Infections		Speech Problem	
Heart Disease		Whooping Cough	

ALLERGIES   YEAR   COMMENTS
- Aspirin
- Bee Sting Requiring Treatment
- Food, Pollens
- Other Medication

Other significant illness, accidents, operations, limitations, and medications.

MEDICAL EXAMINATIONS
Give dates, name of physician and pertinent findings.
C.H.D.P. Complete Exam ☐   Waiver ☐

Mo/Yr	COMMENTS

VISION
CODE: ✓ 20/20   Numerical Figure Represents Vision at 20

	Without Glasses			With Glasses		
Date	Gr.	R	L	R	L	
	P					
	K					
	1					
	2					
	3					
	4					
	5					
	6					
	7					
	8					
	9					
	10					
	11					
	12					

TITMUS SCREENER
- Plus Sphere R
- Plus Sphere L
- Muscle Balance Far
- Muscle Balance Near
- Color Vision
- Binocular Vision

CODE: · Pass − Fail

REMARKS

HEARING
CODE:
√ Normal   P Puretone
F.T. Failed Test   I Impedance
M.U. Mobile Unit   Audiometry
Th Threshold

Date	Gr.	R	L
	P		
	K		
	1		
	2		
	3		
	4		
	5		
	6		
	7		
	8		
	9		
	10		
	11		
	12		

DENTAL SCREENING
Screener RN, DDS, DH

Grade												
Mo/Yr												
Passed												
Immediate Care Needed												
Visible Decay												
Gum Disease												
Orthodontic Problem												
Other Mouth Problems												
Needs Better Brushing & Flossing												

Available from K/P Graphics, Roseville, California.

79

COMMENTS: _____

GIRLS: 2 TO 18 YEARS
PHYSICAL GROWTH
NCHS PERCENTILES*

BOYS: 2 TO 18 YEARS
PHYSICAL GROWTH
NCHS PERCENTILES*

*Adapted from Hamil PVV, Drizd TA, Johnson CL, Reed RB, Roche AF, Moore WM. Physical growth: National Center for Health Statistics percentiles. AM J CLIN NUTR 32:607-629 1979. Data from the National Center for Health Statistics (NCHS), Hyattsville, Maryland. © 1982 ROSS LABORATORIES

Provided as a service of Ross Laboratories

Available from K/P Graphics, Roseville, California.

80

HEALTH RECORD

Final check by nurse | | | | | | | |

ID # _____

Name _____ M _____   Address _____
        Last   First   Middle   F   Birthdate   Phone _____

Father's name _____ Mother's name _____   Lives with _____

Limiting Health Problems				Immunizations	Dates						Father's health Occupation	
						1st	2nd	B	B	B		
Allergy/asthma		Vision									Mother's health Occupation	
Cardiac		Hearing loss		Diphtheria/tetanus							Number siblings	
Diabetes		Orthopedic		Polio							Familial disorders	
Seizure disorder				Measles Rubeola							Other family history	
				Rubella								
				Mumps								
				Other								
				Verifying physician								

Physical Progress Record

Grade		Pre-K	K	1	2	3	4	5	6	7	8	9	10	11	12
Date screened															
School name															
Dental															
ENT															
Height															
Weight															
Nutrition															
Ortho															
Coordination															
Skin-scalp															
Vision	R	20/	20/	20/	20/	20/	20/	20/	20/	20/	20/	20/	20/	20/	20/
Test	L	20/	20/	20/	20/	20/	20/	20/	20/	20/	20/	20/	20/	20/	20/
Vision	R	20/	20/	20/	20/	20/	20/	20/	20/	20/	20/	20/	20/	20/	20/
Glasses	L	20/	20/	20/	20/	20/	20/	20/	20/	20/	20/	20/	20/	20/	20/
Date of vision test															
Color test															
Plus lens															
Hirschberg															
Speech/voice															
B/P															
Nurse/nurse aide name															
Hearing	R														
	L														
Date															
Hearing technician name															

Code—No defect noted; defect noted; corrected; X not correctable; referred.

Physician's Examination

Date				
School				
Sp. ed./UIL/other				
Skin-scalp				
Eyes				
ENT				
Heart				
BP				
Chest				
Lymph nodes				
Abdomen				
Musculoskeletal				
Reflexes/neuro.				
Gen. cond./nutr.				
Examiner				
Dental examination				
Dentist				

Recommendations and restrictions

Program adjustment				
Adaptive P.E.				
UIL X ray				
1.2 Initiated				
Special ed./placement				

HEALTH RECORD
Page 2

Progress Notes

At Beginning of Note, Code Activity—T.N.C., teacher-nurse conference; H.V., home visit; T.V., telephone visit; S.C., student conference. Sign all notes.

Date	Notes	Date	Notes	Date	Notes

SCHOOL HEALTH RECORD

Information Concerning Home

Parent or guardian	Home address (pencil)	Phone	Business address (pencil)	Phone	Family physician (pencil)	
Father					Name	Phone
Mother					Address	

Friend/Relative to Call in Case of Emergency (pencil)

Name	Phone	Name	Phone	Name	Phone
Address		Address		Address	

		Grade																
		Month/year																
Height																		
Weight																		
Visual acuity		B																
		R																
		L																
With glasses		B																
		R																
		L																
Visual acuity (recheck)		B																
		R																
		L																
With glasses		B																
		R																
		L																
Farsightedness																		
BV far																		
BV near																		
Depth perception																		
Color deficient																		
Hearing		R																
		L																
Hearing (recheck)		R																
		L																
Dental status	Good																	
	Needs care																	
Sickle cell (1 X only)																		
Hgb or hematocrit																		
Blood pressure																		
Scoliosis																		
TB skin test (mm)																		

SCHOOL HEALTH RECORD
Page 2

			Month	Day	Year	M F	
Last name		First	Middle	Date of birth	Sex	Race	

Immunization	Dates					Medical history	Date
	1	2	3	Boosters		Allergy and asthma	
DTP						Convulsive disorders	
Td						Crippling conditions	
Tetanus						Chest conditions	
OPV						Chickenpox	
Measles						Diabetes	
Rubella						Eye, ear, nose disease	
Mumps						Heart condition	
Other						Measles	

Comments

Special tests	Date	Results
Cocci		
Histo		
Cholesterol		

Medical history	Date
German measles	
Mumps	
Rheumatic fever	
Strep inf. or scarlet fever	
Tonsillitis	
Valley fever	
Whooping cough	
Operations:	
Serious injury or accident	
Tuberculosis or contact	
Other	

Mo/yr		Active problems	Date resolved
	1		
	2		
	3		
	4		
	5		
	6		
	7		
	8		
	9		
	10		
	11		
	12		
	13		
	14		

Physical assessment				
Date				
Eyes				
Nose				
Teeth				
Gums				
Throat				
Tonsils				
Ears				
Glands				
Heart				
Lungs				
Abdomen				
Hernia				
Orthopedic				
Skin				
Posture				
Nutrition				
Blood pressure				
Speech				
Phys. ed. rec.				

PERMANENT CUMULATIVE HEALTH RECORD

Parent fill in Sections 1, 2, and 3 only

1. Student's name _____ Date of birth _____ M____ F____

      Last   First   M.I.

2. Parent's name _____ Address (in pencil) _____ Phone _____

3. Tag for special health condition _____

Growth Record and Vision

	Year		Year	Date															
Accident—serious		Neurological disorder		Grade															
Allergy—drug/other		Orthopedic handicap		Age															
Asthma		Otitis media		Height															
Blood disorder		Rheumatic fever		Weight															
Cardiac disease/problem		Seizure disorder		Head circumference															
Congenital deformity		Speech disorder		Type of test															
Diabetes		Surgery—serious		Without	R	20/	20/	20/	20/	20/	20/	20/	20/	20/	20/	20/	20/	20/	20/
Hearing loss		T.B. Contact		correction	L	20/	20/	20/	20/	20/	20/	20/	20/	20/	20/	20/	20/	20/	20/
Hypertension		Ulcer		Both eyes		20/	20/	20/	20/	20/	20/	20/	20/	20/	20/	20/	20/	20/	20/
Illness—serious		Urinary problem		With correction	R	20/	20/	20/	20/	20/	20/	20/	20/	20/	20/	20/	20/	20/	20/
Kidney disorder		Vision loss		(glasses or contacts)	L	20/	20/	20/	20/	20/	20/	20/	20/	20/	20/	20/	20/	20/	20/
Muscular disorder		Other																	

Immunization Record

Physician Recommendations, Restrictions, Medications

Hypertension Screening

Prevention Record	Dose 1 Mo/yr	Dose 2 Mo/yr	Dose 3 Mo/yr	Booster Mo/yr	Booster Mo/yr	Reason	Dates				Date				
Diphtheria/pertussis/ tetanus											R				
											L				
Tetanus/diphtheria															

Special Services: Recommendations, Reports, Program Adjustment

Prevention Record															
Polio															
Rubeola (vac. or date/illness)															
Rubella															
Mumps (vac. or date/illness)															
MMR															
TB test															
Chest x ray															
Other															
Verifying physician/clinic															
Nurse/signature															

Medical/religious exemption: _____

Dental Screening*

Date	Results	Referred	Corrected	Rechecked

*C, caries; G, gingivitis; H, hygiene; O, orthodontic; O.K., no problem
All referrals in red ink.

PERMANENT CUMULATIVE HEALTH RECORD
Page 2

Name _____ D.O.B. _____

Teacher Observation

Instructions: Use X when defect observed, circle X when corrected. H.I.—Record health inventory in first TNC column.

Audiometric Screening

Teacher-Nurse Conference Data		HI									Date	Referral and Follow-up	Nurse		Date	Sweep Norm	Audiogram Freq.	250	500	1,000	2,000	3,000	4,000	5,000
General	Tires easily															R	R db							
	Under or overweight															L	L db							
	Posture															R	R db							
	Muscular coordination															L	L db							
	Hair, scalp, skin															R	R db							
	Personal hygiene															L	L db							
Eyes	Eyelids															R	R db							
	Strabismus															L	L db							
	Squint															R	R db							
	Frequent headaches															L	L db							
	Eyes water															R	R db							
Ears	Discharge															L	L db							
	Earaches															R	R db							
	Does not hear well															L	L db							
Nose	Frequent colds—nosebleeds															R	R db							
Mouth	Mouth breathing															L	L db							
Throat	Frequent sore throat																							
	Oral hygiene																							
Teeth	Obvious defects																							
	Gums																							
Behavior Pattern	Disturbs classroom																							
	Nervous/restless																							
	Twitching—fainting																							
	Nail biting																							
	Shy																							
	Overaggressiveness																							
	Frequent stomachaches																							
	Excessive use of toilet																							
	Peer relations																							
	Doesn't like school																							
Other	Food habits																							
	Speech problem																							
	General cleanliness																							
	Excessive absence																							

Scoliosis Screening

Date	Key	Finding/Correction	Nurse

P, passed; Re-Ck; F, failed; R, referred.
All referrals in red ink.

NURSE'S NOTES

Student's name _____

D.O.B. _____

Date		Signature/Title

FORMS FOR
HISTORY OF HEALTH
AND DEVELOPMENT

HEALTH HISTORIES

A health history is rarely a mandatory requirement prior to school entrance. However, it is helpful in the care of many children, especially those with chronic illness or developmental disability.

Several forms are presented in this section. Some are short for specific purposes; others are more detailed. Some are for parents to complete; others are used in a parent-nurse conference.

In some school districts, these forms are developed and used by special education departments. However, many children with chronic health problems such as epilepsy and asthma do not have any educational handicaps, but they do have health problems during school hours, so a good medical history helps in their care.

The history can be written in prose format, as is usually done in a doctor's office or hospital admission, or it can be recorded on a check-off sheet.

Use of the prose format by nonhealth professionals requires some inservice training and a good bit of supervised experience. A good health history is one of the most important components needed for making plans regarding the student's education and health.

The Parent's Medical History: Prenatal and Early Life stresses maternal factors prior to, during and shortly after pregnancy that may (at time of this history recording) influence the student's learning and/or behavior.

The third health history shown should be completed by parents of students entering kindergarten or first grade or who are new to the district. The input by the parent is reviewed by the nurse and recorded on the student's health record when necessary. The information should be considered a supplement to the nurse-parent conference.

At the bottom of the form is a mention of Early Periodic Screening Diagnosis and Treatment (EPSDT). This is a federal program that reimburses health care providers. Some school districts perform these screening exams and are reimbursed from federal funds (Title XIX, Medicaid).

MEDICAL HISTORY UPDATE

The "Medical History Update" is used when a detailed medical history has already been taken and only a brief update is needed.

PARENTS' MEDICAL HISTORY: PRENATAL AND EARLY LIFE

To parents of _____. Please make a ___✓___ over any number or letter for which the answer is "Yes." If the answer is "No," leave the letter or number blank.

Example: If you have had high blood pressure, make a check mark as follows: ✓ High blood pressure.

During Pregnancy

A. Did you have
1. Heart disease?
2. High blood pressure?
3. Edema (swelling) legs or arms?
4. Convulsions?
5. Kidney or bladder infections?
6. Female trouble?

B. Did you
1. Take *any* medication or drugs?
2. Have any illnesses or anemia during pregnancy?

C. Have you had any trauma (physical injury) during this pregnancy?

D. Any emotional stress?

E. Do you use *any* alcohol or tobacco?

F. Did any doctor tell you about any problem with your female organs or pelvis?

G. Have you had
1. Five or more children?
2. Sickle cell disease?
3. Any bleeding or cramping?
4. Premature rupture of the membranes (bag of water)?

H. Have you *ever* had
1. Diabetes or thyroid trouble?
2. Any gland surgery?

I. Have you *ever* had
1. Stillborn children?
2. Miscarriages?
3. Babies that needed an exchange transfusion?
4. Babies born later than 42 weeks (10 months, 2 weeks)?
5. Any premature babies?
6. Babies that died in first month of life?
7. A Caeserean section?
8. Baby born weighing more than 10 pounds?
9. Epilepsy?

PARENTS' MEDICAL HISTORY: PRENATAL AND EARLY LIFE
Page 2

Intra Partum Factors
(shortly before and during labor)

1. Excess fluid in bag of waters?
2. Premature rupture of membranes longer than 12 hours before delivery?
3. Excess sedation?
4. Were you awake during labor?
5. How long did this labor last:
    Less than 5 hours?
    5 to 10 hours?
    10 to 20 hours?
    More than 20 hours?
6. Were you given medicine or a shot to start or strengthen labor?
7. Was the baby born properly and easily or was it difficult?
8. Was it head first, face first, or breech?
9. Were you awake during delivery?

Postnatal Factors
(first week or two of life)

1. Was the baby premature or postmature (more or less than 38 to 42 weeks)?
2. Did baby breathe immediately or need to be made to cry?
3. Was baby under 5 pounds or over 10 pounds?
4. Did baby have any
    Blood problems or jaundice?
    Breathing problems?
    Blue spells?
    Convulsions?
    Need an incubator and oxygen?
5. Did baby suck well in first few days of life?
6. What did baby weigh at birth _____? at age 1 month _____?
7. Did baby have colic—how long did it last?

School _____

Grade _____

Dear Parent:

We would like for your child to gain the most from his/her school experience. In order for us to assist in accomplishing this, it is necessary to have a current health history. Please complete this form and return it to the principal or nurse.

YOUR SCHOOL NURSE

Pupil's Name _____ Sex _____ Birth Date _____
                    (Last)   (First)   (Middle)

Address _____ Phone _____

Father's Name _____ Mother's Name _____

Brothers _____ Sisters _____ This child is _____ in family.
            (Number)   (Number)   (Number)

1. How is health care provided for this student?   Employment Insurance ☐

   Private Insurance ☐   Social Security Insurance ☐   Medicaid ☐   Other ☐ _____

2. With whom does child live? _____

3. When did your child have a physical examination? _____ _____
                                                         Date   Physician/Clinic

   Purpose of examination: Routine check up ☐   Illness/Injury ☐ _____
                                                                           Specify

4. Does your child have a health problem (check where appropriate)

   Asthma _____   Diabetes _____   Vision _____   Sickle Cell Anemia _____   Injury _____

   Allergies _____   Anemia _____   Hearing _____   Seizures/Convulsions _____   Heart _____

   Other _____

5. Does your child take medication? _____ Name of medication(s) _____
                                       Yes/No

6. During the pregnancy with this child, did his mother have any medical problems?
   (e.g., High blood pressure or kidney infection, exposure to other infections.) _____

7. During the pregnancy with this child, did the mother smoke cigarettes? _____ Amount _____.

   Drink alcohol? _____ Amount _____. Take any medication other than vitamins or iron? _____

   Name of medication(s) _____.

8. Were there any problems during labor and delivery? _____ Comments _____

   How long did the labor last? _____ Did the child breathe right away? _____ Birth Weight _____

   How long did the child remain in the hospital after birth? _____

   Did the child leave the hospital when his/her mother left? _____

   What age did your child: Walk alone? _____ Talk (2 words together)? _____ Daytime toilet trained? _____

   Is bedwetting a problem? _____ If so, explain _____

9. Has child been hospitalized for any reason since birth? _____

10. Does any close relative in your family have a history of: (Check and indicate relationship to this child.)
    Diabetes _____   Cancer _____   High Blood Pressure _____   Birth Defect _____
    Anemia _____   Epilepsy _____   Sickle Cell Anemia _____   Heart Disease _____
    Learning Problems _____   Mental Retardation _____   Other _____

11. Are there any problems in the home which might affect your child's learning? _____ Comment: _____

12. Is there anything more about this child's health that you think is important for us to know? _____

    Explain: _____

_____ _____ Date _____
         Parent's Signature

    Independent School District is certified to provide EPSDT (Early Periodic Screening Diagnosis and Treatment) screening.

93

HISTORIA CLINICA

_____
Escuela

_____
Grado

Estimados Padres:

Nos gustaría que su niño/a lograra el máximo de sus experiencias en la escuela. Para que nosotros podamos ayudarlo a lograr esto, es necesario tener una completa historia clínica al corriente. Por favor, completar esta forma y regreselo al Director o la enfermera de la escuela.

SU ENFERMERA ESCOLAR

Nombre del Alumno _____ Sexo _____ Fecha de nacimento _____
(Apellido del padre)   _(Nombre)_   _(Apellido de la madre)_

Dirección _____ Número de Teléfono _____

Nombre del Padre _____ Nombre de la Madre _____

Hermanos _____ Hermanas _____ Este niño/a es _____ en la familia.
(Número de)   _(Número de)_   _(El Número)_

1. ¿Tiene usted lo segúiente para su niño/a? Seguran za de su Compañia ☐

   Segurancia Privado ☐   Segurancia de Seguro Social ☐   Medicaid ☐   Otro ☐ _____

2. ¿Con quién vive el niño/a? _____

3. ¿Cuando fué la última vez que su niño/a recibio un examen físico? _____ _____
   Fecha   _Médico/Clínica_

   Razón del examen: Examen rutina ☐   Enfermedad/Herido ☐ _____
   Explique

4. ¿Tiene su niño/a una problema de salud? (Marcar donde es propio)

   Asma _____   Diabetes _____   Problemas de la vista _____   Drepanocito (sickle cell) _____   Herido _____

   Alergias _____   Anemia _____   Problemas del oido _____   Ataques/convulsiónes _____

   Enfermedad del corazón _____   Otro _____

5. ¿Toma su niño/a medicina(s)? _____ Nombre de medicina(s) _____
   _Si/No_

6. ¿Durante su embarazo, con este/a niño/a, tuvo la madre problemas de salud? _____
   (e.g., alta presión o infección del riñón, infecciones contagiosas)

7. Durante su embarazo con esteá niño/a fumó, cigarillos? _____ Cantidad _____

   Tomó bebidas alcohólicas _____ Cantidad _____ . Tomó medicina(s) aparte de vitaminas

   o hierro? _____ Nombre de medicina(s) _____

8. ¿Tuvo problemas durante su parto? _____ Comentario _____

   ¿Cuánto tiempo duró su parto? _____ ¿Respiro el niño immediatamente? _____ Peso al nacer _____

   ¿Cuánto tiempo duro el niño/a en la hospital después de nacimiento? _____

   ¿Se fué el niño/a para la casa con la mamá? _____

   ¿A que edad: caminó solo su niño/a? _____ ¿Habló dos palabras en junto? _____

   ¿A que edad empezó usar el laboratorio? _____

   ¿Se moja la cama? Si su repuesta es si, por favor explicar. _____

9. ¿Ha sido niño/a admitido en un hospital por alguna razón desde nacimiento? _____

10. ¿Alguna persona en su familia tiene historia de: (Marque quién.)
    Diabetes _____   Cancer _____   Presión alta _____   Defecto de nacimiento _____
    Anemia _____   Epilepsia/Ataques _____   Drepanocito _____   Enfermedad del Corazón _____
    Problemas de aprender _____   Retardación _____   Otro _____

11. ¿Hay problemas en su casa que podrán afectar el progreso de su niño/a? _____

    Comentario: _____

12. Nos puede decir algo de importancia de la salud de su niño/a que nosotros no le hayamos preguntado? _____

_____ Fecha _____
Firma del Padre

Independent School District esta certificardo para dar EPSDT (Evaluación Primaria de Diagnoses y Tratamiento) examenaciónes.

COMPREHENSIVE HEALTH HISTORY
(NURSE/PARENT CONFERENCE)

I. Student profile

Name _____

Date _____ Age _____

D.O.B. _____ Sex: M F

Grade _____

School _____

Date of history _____

Recorder _____

Informant _____

Interviewer _____

Health care provider _____

Medicaid: No   Yes _____
Number

II. Referred for evaluation of (circle)   Referred by _____
Relationship to pupil

  A. Low academic progress or academic problem

  B. Attention deficit

  C. Hyperactivity

  D. Behavior

  E. Related health problem(s)

  F. Developmental delay

  G. Other

III. Health problem(s), during past 12 months (list and describe management/treatment). Are there other known health problems?

IV. Past history (list with date and age):

  A. Hospitalizations—(include reason)—overnight stay, emergency room visit, outpatient, day surgery?

  B. Illness (including contagious diseases, high fever, etc.)?

  C. Injuries—accidents, ingestions, head injury, sequale?

  D. Medications?

  E. Allergies?

  F. Last health care visit _____ Name of provider _____

   Purpose of visit: acute care? routine P.E.? _____

   Dental care   Date of last visit _____ Purpose _____ Provider _____

  G. Prenatal: Maternal age _____ Length of pregnancy _____ # of pregnancy _____
   # of living children _____ # of miscarriages _____ Prenatal care (where and what month begun) _____ Habits   (circle): smoking, drinking, drugs, pica, other _____
   (Explain) _____
   High risks   (circle): Infections, bleeding, high blood pressure, anemia, fever, RH factor, trauma, inherited disease(s), medications, weight gain, chronic disease, hospitalization, other _____

   _____

   _____

COMPREHENSIVE HEALTH HISTORY
(NURSE/PARENT CONFERENCE)
Page 2

Name _____

H. Labor and delivery
1. Place _____
2. Length of labor _____
3. Type of delivery _____
4. Condition of mother _____
5. Problems (circle): breathing, forceps, C-section, other _____
6. Birth weight _____

I. Neonatal
Problems (circle): breathing, infections, RH factor, jaundice, transfusions, bleeding, congenital anomaly, feeding, other _____

J. Postnatal
Mother home from hospital in _____ days.
Baby home in _____ days. Complications? Explain. _____
_____

K. Development (state age, if known)
1. Sat alone	4. Walked alone	7. Other (Big Wheel _____,
2. Crawled	5. Combined words	_____ roller skated, etc.)
3. Stood	6. Toilet trained	8. School performance

Development is (circle) faster, slower, equal to siblings or peers?
Comments:

V. Family history
Biological mother: Age _____ Health _____

Biological father: Age _____ Health _____

Siblings: Name   Sex Age   Health
1. _____
2. _____
3. _____
4. _____

Maternal grandparents   Paternal grandparents

GM Age _____ Health _____   GM Age _____ Health _____

GF Age _____ Health _____   GF Age _____ Health _____

Family diseases (circle): Heart disease, stroke, hypertension, diabetes, asthma, allergy, anemia, sickle cell disease or trait, arthritis, cancer, epilepsy, cataracts, glaucoma, kidney disease, tuberculosis, mental problems, mental retardation, learning problems, other. Explain.

VI. Social history
A. Household members?
B. Housing?
C. Others caring for child:?

COMPREHENSIVE HEALTH HISTORY
(NURSE/PARENT CONFERENCE)
Page 3

Name _____

VII. Habits (sleep, thumb sucking, nightmares, sleepwalking, rocking)?

VIII. Any problems parent or child wishes to discuss?

IX. Review of systems (circle)

1. General—Changes in weight, appetite, activity level, bowel habits, resistance to disease, other. (Explain.) Birth defects—congenital anomalies.

2. Skin—Rashes, easy bruising, changes in skin color or texture, eczema, impetigo, growths, or tumors. (Explain.)

3. Head—Headache, trauma, infections. (Explain.)

4. Eyes—Vision changes, trauma, infections, cataracts, glaucoma, other. (Explain.)

5. Ears, nose, throat—Infections (specify), trauma, epistaxis, allergies, hearing changes, voice changes, caries, speech problems. (Explain.)

6. Neck—Trauma, swollen lymph nodes, limitation of movement. (Explain.)

7. Respiratory—Infections, breathing problems, trauma, wheezing, cough, asthma. (Explain.)

8. Cardiovascular—Murmur, fatigue with exertion, cyanosis. (Explain.)

9. Gastrointestinal—Abdominal pain, nausea, jaundice, vomiting, diarrhea, constipation, ulcer. (Explain.)

10. Genitourinary—Infections, enuresis, encopresis, discharge, rashes, menstruation, sexual development. (Explain.)

11. Musculoskeletal—Trauma, limitation of movement, joint pain or swelling, growths or tumor, curvature of the spine, braces, corrective shoes. (Explain.)

12. Neurological—Birth injury, trauma, seizures (febrile versus afebrile), staring spells, poor coordination or balance, dizziness, syncope, developmental evaluation. (Explain.)

13. Endocrine—Increased thirst, appetite, urination, diabetes, thyroid problems. (Explain.)

14. Hematologic—Anemia, blood transfusions, blood dyscrasias, sickle cell. (Explain.)

15. Psychosocial—Changes in activity level, behavior, relationships, punishment, rewards (Explain.)

16. Nutrition—(24-hour recall including snacks).

Name _____

X. Summary of pertinent history (list in priority)

    A.

    B.

    C.

    D.

    E.

    F.

XI. Records request(s)

    A.

    B.

    C.

    D.

XII. Physical examination (circle one)

    A. Has been requested from physician or health care facility.

    B. On file, see attached current medical records.

    C. Needed, refer to private physician due to _____

    D. Needed, schedule exam by _____

HISTORY—SCHOOL HEALTH SERVICES

SS #: _____

Medicaid No.: _____

ID no.: _____

Name of child _____ Date _____

D.O.B. _____ Age _____ Sex: M F Ethnic group _____

Home address _____ Zip _____ Phone number _____

School _____ Grade _____

Reason for exam ☐ Special education ☐ Health care maintenance ☐ EPSDT

☐ _____

Informant(s) _____

Current Problems (Health, Behavior, and/or Academic: List and describe; be specific.)

Past history	Family/social history
Prenatal/birth	
Neonatal	
Growth and development	
Behavior	
School performance problems	
Immunizations	**Review of systems**
Test	
Illnesses/hospitalizations	
Allergies	
Medications	

Physical Examination

Name of child _____ Date of examination _____

Height		Weight		Vision					Hearing		
				Without glasses		**With glasses**			**Right**		**Left**
in.		lb.									
cm.		kg.		Right	Left	Right	Left				
% ile		% ile		20/	20/	20/	20/		Method Used:		

Instructions: Describe fully any abnormal findings.

B.P. _____ Head circumference: _____ cm

P _____ R _____ (_____% ile)

	Normal	Abnormal	Not Examined	
General				
Appearance				
Skin				
HEENT				
Head				
Ears				
Eyes				
Nose/throat				
Mouth/teeth				
Chest/lungs				
Cardiovascular				
Abdomen				
Genitalia				
Extremities joints/spine				
Neurological Onentation				
Behavior				
Cerebellar function				
Sensory				
Motor				
Reflexes				
Cranial nerves				
Developmental assessment				

Name of child _____ Date of examination _____

Medical impression/problem list:

Recommendations/anticipatory guidance:

Current medication:

Educational implications: ☐ Yes ☐ No (Will findings influence learning; require special equipment or an adjustment in the school program environment?)

Explanation:

Follow-up needed: _____ Date: _____ By whom? _____

Laboratory results:

Signed: _____

_____
Title

_____
Name printed

_____
Address

_____
Zip code   Telephone

MEDICAL HISTORY UPDATE

Date _____

Name _____ Birthdate _____

School _____ Grade _____ Special class _____

Last complete medical evaluation _____
                                        Date

Last update of developmental history _____
                                              Date

Significant illnesses, accidents, and/or medical problems since last evaluated

_____

_____

_____

_____

_____

Present medical problems _____

_____

Current medications _____

_____

Changes in socioeconomic conditions since last evaluated _____

_____

Vision: R _____ L _____ Hearing: R _____ L _____ Height _____ Weight _____

Dental _____

_____
School nurse

REQUEST FOR HEALTH INFORMATION

To: _____
       School   _____
                                                              Address

_____   _____
       Physician or clinic

_____   _____
       Address with zip   Pupil's name

                                                              _____
                                                              Address with zip

                                                              _____
                                                              School   Birthdate

Instructions: We would appreciate your answering the items
checked below to help us plan the best school program for   _____
this pupil for these reasons: Father's name

                                                              _____
                                                              Mother's name

_____

_____

_____

Date of request _____

                                        Thank you,

                                        _____ School nurse, R.N.

_____

_____ **Diagnosis?** _____

_____ **Is treatment completed?** _____

_____ **X-ray findings?** _____

_____ **Should pupil have limited physical activities, how limited, and for how long?**
_____

_____

_____ **Any other suggestions for this child's program at school?** _____

_____

_____

_____   _____
       Date of this report   Signature of physician

_____

Consent

I authorize and request _____ **through its authorized employees to furnish to**

_____
Last name   First name   Number   Street   City   State   Zip code

the transcribed medical findings of the evaluation on _____
                                                                          Patient's name

_____   _____
   Date   Signature of legal guardian   Witness

103

STUDENT HEALTH APPRAISAL FOR DRIVER TRAINING

Student's name _____

Date of birth _____

School _____ Grade _____

Date _____

1. Does your son or daughter have any impairments or health conditions that would limit or create difficult or dangerous situations in a behind-the-wheel Driver Training class? (Please check) ( ) heart ( ) fainting ( ) orthopedic ( ) diabetes ( ) epilepsy ( ) allergic reactions	If the answer is yes to any of these, please explain. If episodes of feeling faint, dizzy, or confused, give the number of episodes in past three years and the date of last occurrence.
2. Is your son or daughter currently receiving medication or under a doctor's care?	If the answer is yes, please explain.
3. Does your son or daughter have any vision or hearing problems?	If the answer is yes, please explain.
4. Are there any indications that your son or daughter has an emotional or physical condition that might create problems as a result of Driver Training?	If the answer is yes, please explain.

5. Are there any other comments or recommendations you might have?

_____

I affirm that the above statements are true to the best of my knowledge.

_____ _____
Parent's signature

_____

Referral to the Nurse for Review

Vision satisfactory? _____ Yes _____ No

Hearing satisfactory? _____ Yes _____ No

Comments _____

_____

_____

_____
Nurse's signature

FORMS FOR HEARING SCREENINGS AND TESTING

HEARING SCREENING REPORT FOR SCHOOL YEAR

The Hearing Screening Report for School Year is to be used for comprehensive monthly or annual reports. It may be submitted to the central health office, the state health department, or the education agency.

Here are the instructions for completing the form:

1. Name of School or District—self-explanatory.
2. County—self-explanatory.
3. Reported by (name of person making the report).
4. Title (title of the person making the report).
5. Date—self-explanatory.

Column A: Number of children screened for hearing problems.

Column B: Number of children referred to a physician.

Column C: Number of children listed in column B who *were not* seen by a physician, or information unknown.

Column D: Number of children listed in column B who *were* seen by a physician.

Each column is listed by the grade in which the child is enrolled. Special education children should be listed separately *if* they are screened separately. Columns C and D should equal column B; columns E, F, and G should equal column D.

Column E: Number of children listed in column D who had no problem upon medical examination by a physician.

Column F: Number of children listed in column D who were examined and no treatment prescribed.

Column G: Number of children listed in column D who received treatment from a physician.

HEARING SCREENING: AUDIOGRAM RECORD

While most schools utilize school nurses, audiologists, or language pathologists to do audiograms, some use volunteers. All school hearing screeners should take an approved course (usually state mandated) and be required to demonstrate proficiency.

Most school nurses perform "sweep-check" audiograms: 20–25 decibels at 500, 1,000, 2,000, and 4,000 Hertz.

If the child fails the sweep-check, a complete audiogram should be done at levels up to 80 to 100 decibels. The form should be filled out and given to the parent to take to the child's ear specialist.

The Hearing Screening: Audiogram Record is used to record results of audiometric examination. An inservice workshop is required to be able to perform the audiometric exam and complete the form.

LIST OF PUPILS GIVEN HEARING THRESHOLD TESTS AND FOLLOW-UP INFORMATION

The hearing screener uses the following form to record results of that day's screening. When screen has been completed on that campus for all the children who require it, the results are usually entered onto the student's permanent record card and the appropriate physician/audiologist referrals are made by the hearing screener.

ANNUAL/MONTHLY HEARING REPORT

The Annual/Monthly Hearing Report records the total number of students screened on each campus. It can be submitted as a monthly or annual report.

RESULTS FROM ELECTROACOUSTIC IMPEDANCE AUDIOMETRY

At this time, most medical authorities agree that the impedance bridge should not be used as a substitute for audiometric screening. While it is admittedly difficult to screen 4- and 5-year-old children by regular screening audiometry, with patience and skill, most can be validly screened.

Most otologists do not currently recommend the impedance bridge for mass screening of large numbers of asymptomatic children. Most abnormal impedance bridge results are due to asymptomatic middle ear effusion (serous otitis media) that improves in 6 to 12 weeks with no treatment. If tympanometric screening is performed, it should always be repeated in 12 weeks for all children who failed the first time, prior to referral. Referral to a physician without rescreening often results in needless treatment and expense for the family.

If, following audiometric screening and direct visualization of the eardrum with an otoscope, the school nurse suspects serous otitis media, impedance bridge audiometry can help to confirm the diagnosis prior to referral to the pediatrician or ear specialist.

The Results from Electroacoustic Impedance Audiometry is completed by the audiologist. If a child with an ear problem is referred to a physician, this form (plus the audiogram) should save the parent the expense of having it repeated in the doctor's office.

HEARING SCREENING REPORT FOR SCHOOL YEAR

Name of school or district _____ County _____

Reported by _____ Title _____ Date _____

Columns C + D = B; Columns E + F + G = D.

Grades	Number of children screened.	Number of Column A who were referred to a physician.	Number of Column B not seen by a physician (or information unknown).	Number of Column B who were seen by a physician.	Number of Column D were examined; no problem found.	Number of Column D who were examined; no treatment prescribed.	Number of Column D who were examined and treated.	Did you also screen for vision problems? Yes ____ No ____. If "Yes", please complete separate form.
		A	B	C	D	E	F	G
Preschool								
Special Ed.								
K								
1								
2								
3								
4								
5								
6								
7								
8								
9								
10								
11								
12								
Subtotals				C	D	E	F	G

Total of C + D = B   Total of E + F + G = D

Totals	A		B	C	D	E	F	G

Please note that column totals must balance and equal.
Referral criteria: *Signs & Symptoms* or failure to respond to two of the four frequencies: 500, 1,000, 2,000, and 4,000 Hz in either ear at 25 dB ANSI.

HEARING CONSERVATION PROGRAM REPORT

School name _____   District _____

Address _____   Phone _____

Form completed by _____   Date _____

1. Number of students initially screened.   _____
2. Number of students failing first screening.   _____
    A. Number of referrals after first screening.   _____
    B. Number of referrals actually seen.   _____
3. Number of students receiving second screening.   _____
4. Number of students failing second screening.   _____
    A. Number of medical referrals.   _____
    B. Number of referrals actually seen.   _____
    C. Number of audiological referrals.   _____
    D. Number of audiological referrals seen.   _____
    E. Number of students receiving H.A.E.s   _____
5. Number of students receiving "at-risk letters."   _____ (optional)
6. Number of students receiving "noise letters."   _____ (optional)
7. Number of students wearing hearing aids.   _____
8. Number of students failing screening who received special education
    evaluations.   _____

                                    Return to _____

Number of audiometers in school _____

Date of last calibration of equipment _____

ANNUAL REPORT OF HEARING TESTING

School district _____ **Superintendent** _____

Address _____

Period covered _____ **Prepared by** _____
from / to

Office phone (   ) _____

Grades in District (circle highest) (1)	Enter No. Pupils Enrolled in each grade as of October (R-30) Reports (2)	Initial Screening — No. Pupils Screened per Sec. 2951 (d) CAC Title 17 (3)	No. Pupils failed Threshold Tests per Sec. 2951 (g) CAC Title 17 (4)	No. of New Hearing Cases (from 4) (5)	No. of Old Hearing Cases (from 4) (6)	No. Pupils Referred for Medical Evaluation (from 4) (7)	No. Pupils Examined by Doctor or Under Treatment (8)
K or 1							
2							
3							
4							
5							
6							
7							
8							
9							
10 or 11							
12							

Special Education

Describe audiometric and audiologic services provided pupils.

HEARING SCREENING—AUDIOGRAM RECORD

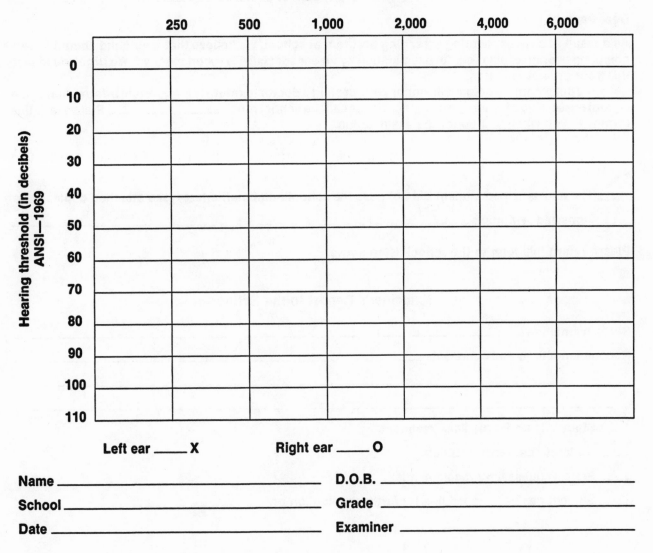

Frequency (in hertz)

Left ear _____ X   Right ear _____ O

Name _____   D.O.B. _____

School _____   Grade _____

Date _____   Examiner _____

HEARING REFERRAL AND REPORT

Student _____

School _____

Dear Parent:

As a result of a recent hearing screening program at school, we believe that your child should have a complete hearing evaluation. An examination by an ear specialist is recommended. We urge you to give this your prompt attention.

Your signature below will authorize your child's doctor to return this important information to the school nurse. If you have any questions, please call the school nurse at _____. Please take this form with you when you go for the examination.

Note to the Examiner: We have directed the parent's attention to the need for a hearing evaluation because

_____ The above-named student did not pass the school audiometric tests (see attached copies).

_____ Signs and symptoms _____

Please return this form to the school listed above.

Examiner's Report to the School

Student's name _____

Recommendations and comments _____

_____

_____

_____ Student is under medical treatment.

_____ No treatment recommended.

_____ Preferential seating recommended.

_____ Student has been scheduled for further evaluation on _____.

Date

_____
Examiner's signature   Date

_____
Address

HEARING SCREENING RECORD FORM

Name _____ Date _____ School _____

Age _____ Grade _____ Teacher _____

Comments from teacher (hearing difficulty, etc.) _____

_____

_____

Sweep Screening

Left: Pass Fail

Right: Pass Fail
   (Circle one)

Comments _____

_____

_____

_____

Threshold 1 Date			Threshold 2 Date		
Freq.	Left	Right	Freq.	Left	Right
250			250		
500			500		
1,000			1,000		
2,000			2,000		
4,000			4,000		

Pass   Fail   (circle one)   Pass   Fail

Comments   Comments

_____

Screener

Notes to Screener

Sweep Screening: 25 dB at 500, 1,000, 2,000, 4,000 Hz.
  Failure to respond to any one frequency constitutes a failure and requires threshold testing.

Threshold tests: For all children who
1. Fail sweep screen.
2. Are referred for further audiological evaluation.

Failure:
1. Hearing level of 30 dB or higher for two or more frequencies in an ear, or a hearing level of 40 dB or higher for any one frequency, on two threshold tests completed at an interval of two weeks.
2. Evidence of pathology (e.g., infection, drainage, or earache).

HIGH-FREQUENCY HEARING LOSS

To the Parents of _____ Date _____

Many children in school have some hearing loss resulting from exposure to loud sounds such as shooting, exploding firecrackers, listening to loud music, driving tractors, driving snowmobiles, working in sawmills, etc. Such hearing loss is permanent and is not treatable medically or surgically.

In most instances, this type of hearing loss does not interfere with the child's ability to hear and understand speech. However, with continued exposure to these noises through the years, this irreversible hearing loss can progress to a level where the understanding of speech is affected, making it difficult for a person to understand clearly what is being said.

Your child's hearing has been tested and found to be well within normal limits for the speech range. However, there is some evidence of depression of hearing at tones immediately above the speech range. This characteristic is frequently related to noise exposure.

It is very important to protect your child's ears from exposure to loud sounds. Earplugs designed for protection against noise should be worn at all times in the presence of excessive noises. Such plugs are inexpensive and are available through your local drugstore.

_____

School nurse

_____

School

LIST OF PUPILS GIVEN HEARING THRESHOLD TESTS AND FOLLOW-UP INFORMATION

School _____

Date _____

Pupil's name	Grade	Room	Reason for threshold test				Results of tests				New case	Old case	Follow-up Information			
			Failed screening	Teacher referral	Previously known	Other	First Test		Final Test				Parent notified	Examined by doctor	Under treatment	No info.
							File, no action	To be requested	File, no action	Follow-up needed						

List the names of all pupils for whom threshold tests are indicated.

115

ANNUAL/MONTHLY HEARING REPORT

Month and year _____   **Name** _____

| | | 1 | 2 | 3 | 4 | 5 | 6 | 7 | 8 | 9 | 10 | 11 | 12 | 13 | 14 | 15 | 16 | 17 | 18 | 19 | 20 | 21 | |
Date	School	Pre school	K	1	2	3	4	5	6	7	8	9	10	11	12	Sp. Ed.	Adult	Total	Pass	Fail	Old loss	New loss	Could not test	I M P
Totals																								

Columns 1 through 16 should equal column 17; column 18 plus column 19 should equal column 17; column 20 plus column 21 should equal column 19.

Nurses/nurse assistants or others testing hearing are to submit completed form monthly to the hearing technician.

RESULTS FROM ELECTROACOUSTIC IMPEDANCE AUDIOMETRY

Name _____ Date _____ Examiner _____

School _____ Grade _____

I. Impedance Data
A. Tympanometry

3.2				3.2
3.1				3.1
2.5				2.5
2.2				2.2
2.1				2.1
1.5				1.5
1.2				1.2
1.1				1.1
0.5				0.5
0.2				0.2
0.1				0.1

−400 −360 −320 −280 −240 −200 −160 −120 −80 −40   0   +40 +80 +120 +160 +200

−20   +20

CC-Equivalent middle ear pressure

B.   CC + 200 mm/H_2O Static compliance

Probe right _____ _____ _____

Probe left _____ _____ _____

C. Acoustic reflex data

Probe right threshold (dB HTL)							
500	1,000	2,000	4,000				
Auditory threshold sensitivity of left ear (dB HTL)							

Probe left threshold (dB HTL)							
500	1,000	2,000	4,000				
Auditory threshold sensitivity of right ear (dB HTL)							

II. Classification of results
(see reverse side for interpretation)

	Right ear	Left ear
Tympanometry (type)		
Static compliance		
Acoustic reflex thresholds		
Pure tone		
Canals		

DNT, did not test; CNT, could not test; NR, no response at limits of equipment; NO, non occlusive; O, occlusive.

Guide for Interpreting Middle Ear Impedance Measurements
(Impedance Audiometry)

I. Tympanometry (pressure/compliance function of the tympanic membrane)

Type A	Ad	Af	B	C
Suggests normal middle ear function	Suggests excessive mobility of the tympanic membrane and ossicular chain (e.g., discontinuity or scarred and atrophic membranes)	Suggests decreased mobility of the tympanic membrane and ossicular chain (ossicular chain fixation)	Suggests little or no mobility of the tympanic membrane (e.g., advanced serous otitis media, adhesive otitis media, cholesteatoma)	Suggests significant negative pressure (less than 150 mm/H_2O in middle ear, cavity

II. Static compliance

	Less than .28 cc*	.29 cc 1.72 cc	1.73 cc (plus)†
	Abnormally low	Normal	Abnormally high

*Abnormally low static compliance is commensurate with decreased mobility of the tympanic membrane and ossicular chain.
†High static compliance is commensurate with excessive mobility of the tympanic membrane and ossicular chain.

III. Stapedial muscle reflex thresholds

Present at all frequencies	Normal hearing*	Mild hearing loss†	Moderate to severe sensorineural hearing loss with recruitment‡	
Absent	Can be absent in some patients with normal hearing	Middle ear pathology	Moderate to severe sensorineural hearing loss without recruitment	Paralysis of cranial VII with normal hearing and no middle ear pathology
Partial	Hearing loss at frequencies reflex is absent			

*The normal threshold is 70–90 dB HL.
†Thresholds range from 95–110 dB HL.
‡Less than 50–60 dB SL.

FORMS FOR HEIGHT AND WEIGHT

WEIGHT-HEIGHT AVERAGES

Weight can be measured on a standard beam balance scale or with a high grade floor model spring scale; they are equally accurate. For perfect accuracy, they must be calibrated annually, but for practical purposes, this is not necessary since the height and weight at any given time is not as important as the *change* over a period of time. Since prepubertal school-age children grow slowly, *monthly* changes will be small. Each year 1 to 2 pounds and 4 to 7 inches are added by most children.

To measure *height,* the measuring rod on a standard balance beam scale is inaccurate. Standing height should be measured against a steel or wood measuring tape fixed to the wall. The head is placed looking straight ahead with chin parallel to the floor. A square block or box or a triangle should be used to extend a line from the top of the child's head to the wall.

The diagnosis of overweight, underweight, or small size is unjustified solely on the basis of height and weight measures. By visual inspection, the child can be classified as grossly overweight, moderately underweight, or grossly underweight. This assessment can be made without knowledge of the actual body weight. In general, most school children in the United States classified as underweight are constitutionally slender rather than malnourished, and most children considered overweight are so because of heredity and excessive caloric intake rather than glandular disease. However, growth charts are convenient for viewing the children's measurements in relation to their peers as well as to their own measurements over a period of years. (See *School Health: A Guide for Health Professionals,* American Academy of Pediatrics, 1981.)

Height-weight grids are useful, but rarely do nurses or aides have time to fill one out for each child. They are simple to use, however:

1. Locate the student's age at the bottom of the page.
2. Locate the weight or height at the side of the page.
3. Where the horizontal and vertical lines intersect, place a dot.
4. Connect dots with a line.

I recommend their use in school only for children with chronic health or nutritional problems.

Head circumference grids are useful for children with spina bifida and/or intracranial shunts and other children who may show abnormal head growth such as microcephaly (excessively small head) or abnormally shaped head.

GROWTH CHARTS

The height, weight, and head circumference grid growth charts for boys and girls are used to detect a deviation from normal growth over prolonged periods of time.

A dot is placed in the proper square each year. Each dot is then connected by a straight line. As long as the line continues to move upward in the same "channel," growth is normal. If the line deviates up or down to a different channel, it is a signal of a possible health problem and should be investigated further.

WEIGHT-HEIGHT AVERAGES

	BOYS				GIRLS			
	PERCENTILES			AGE	PERCENTILES			
	5th	50th	95th	YRS.	5th	50th	95th	
IN.	35	37¼	40¼	3.0	34½	37	39½	IN.
LB.	26½	32¼	39¼		25½	31	38	LB.
IN.	36½	39	41½	3.5	36	38½	41¼	IN.
LB.	28¼	34½	41½		27¼	33¼	41	LB.
IN.	37½	40¼	43¼	4.0	37½	40	42½	IN.
LB.	30	36½	44½		29	35¼	44	LB.
IN.	39	42	44½	4.5	38½	41¼	44	IN.
LB.	31½	39	47½		30½	37	46½	LB.
IN.	40¼	43¼	46	5.0	39½	42½	45½	IN.
LB.	33½	41¼	51		32	39	49½	LB.
IN.	41¼	44½	47¼	5.5	41	44	47	IN.
LB.	35½	43¼	54¼		33½	41	53¼	LB.
IN.	42½	45½	48½	6.0	42	45	48¼	IN.
LB.	37¼	45½	58		35½	43	56½	LB.
IN.	43½	46½	49½	6.5	43	46¼	49½	IN.
LB.	39¼	48	62		37¼	45½	60½	LB.
IN.	44½	48	51	7.0	44	47½	51	IN.
LB.	41	50¼	66½		39	48¼	65½	LB.
IN.	45½	49	52¼	7.5	45	48½	52¼	IN.
LB.	43	53	71¼		41	51¼	70½	LB.
IN.	46½	50	53½	8.0	46	49½	53½	IN.
LB.	45	55½	76		43¼	54½	76½	LB.
IN.	47½	51	54½	8.5	47	51	55	IN.
LB.	47	58½	81½		45½	58½	82½	LB.
IN.	48½	52	55½	9.0	48	52	56¼	IN.
LB.	49	62	87¼		48	62½	89½	LB.
IN.	49¼	53	57	9.5	49¼	53¼	57½	IN.
LB.	51¼	65½	93¼		50½	67¼	96½	LB.
IN.	50¼	54½	58¼	10.0	50¼	54½	58½	IN.
LB.	53½	69¼	99½		53½	71½	104	LB.
IN.	51¼	55¼	59½	10.5	51¼	55½	60¼	IN.
LB.	56¼	73½	106½		56½	76½	111½	LB.
IN.	52¼	56½	61	11.0	52½	57	61½	IN.
LB.	59	77½	113½		60	81½	119	LB.
IN.	53¼	57½	62½	11.5	53½	58½	62½	IN.
LB.	62¼	82½	120½		63½	86½	126½	LB.
IN.	54¼	59	64	12.0	55	59½	64	IN.
LB.	65½	87½	128		67¼	91½	134	LB.
IN.	55¼	60¼	65½	12.5	56¼	60½	65¼	IN.
LB.	69½	93¼	135½		71¼	96½	141¼	LB.
IN.	56¼	61½	66½	13.0	57¼	61½	66¼	IN.
LB.	74¼	99	143¼		75¼	101½	148¼	LB.
IN.	57¼	63	68¼	13.5	58	62½	67	IN.
LB.	79	105½	151		79¼	106½	155	LB.
IN.	58½	64¼	69½	14.0	58½	63¼	67½	IN.
LB.	84¼	112	159		83¼	110½	161	LB.
IN.	59½	65½	70½	14.5	59	63½	67½	IN.
LB.	89½	118½	166½		87	114½	166½	LB.
IN.	61	66½	71½	15.0	59¼	63½	68	IN.
LB.	95	125	174½		90¼	118¼	171½	LB.
IN.	62¼	67½	72½	15.5	59½	63½	68¼	IN.
LB.	100¼	131¼	181½		93¼	121¼	175½	LB.
IN.	63½	68¼	73	16.0	59½	64	68¼	IN.
LB.	105¼	137	188½		95½	123¼	178½	LB.
IN.	64¼	69	73½	16.5	60	64	68¼	IN.
LB.	109½	142	195¼		97½	124½	180½	LB.
IN.	65	69¼	73½	17.0	60	64¼	68¼	IN.
LB.	113½	146¼	201¼		98½	125	181½	LB.
IN.	65¼	69½	73½	17.5	60¼	64¼	68¼	IN.
LB.	116½	149½	206½		99½	125	182¼	LB.
IN.	65¼	69½	73½	18.0	60½	64½	68¼	LB.
LB.	119	151½	211		99½	124½	181½	LB.

WEIGHT CHART—BOYS

Boys: 2 to 18 years
Physical weight growth
NCHS percentiles
Name _____ **Record #** _____

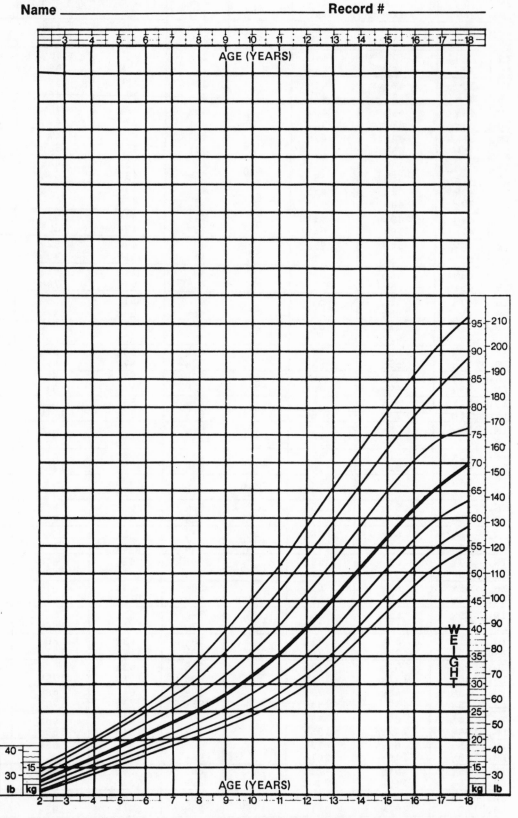

Adapted from data from the National Center for Health Statistics (NCHS) Hyattsville, Maryland.

WEIGHT CHART—GIRLS

Girls: 2 to 18 years
Physical weight growth
NCHS percentiles

Name _____ Record # _____

AGE (YEARS)

AGE (YEARS)

WEIGHT

Adapted from data from the National Center for Health Statistics (NCHS) Hyattsville, Maryland.

HEIGHT CHART—BOYS

Boys: 2 to 18 years
Physical height growth
NCHS percentiles

Name _____ Record # _____

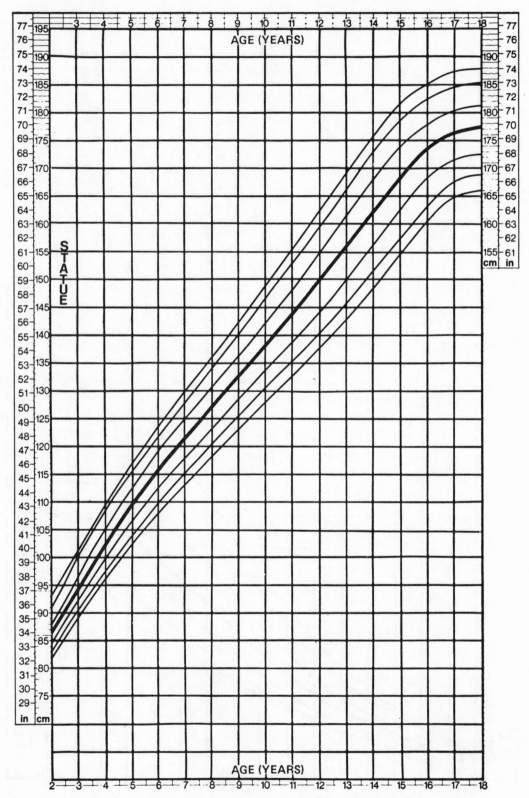

AGE (YEARS)

STATURE

AGE (YEARS)

Adapted from data from the National Center for Health Statistics (NCHS) Hyattsville, Maryland.

HEIGHT CHART—GIRLS

Girls: 2 to 18 years
Physical height growth
NCHS percentiles

Name _____ Record # _____

Adapted from data from the National Center for Health Statistics (NCHS) Hyattsville, Maryland.

HEAD CIRCUMFERENCE—BOYS

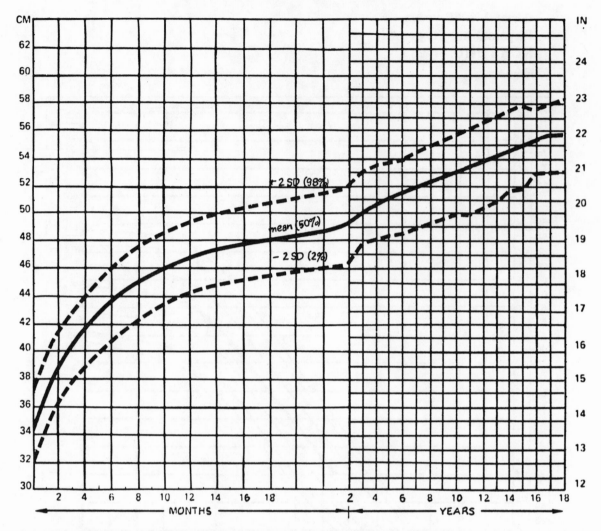

Ref: NELLHAUS, G., Composite International & Interracial Graphs, Pediatrics 41:106, 1968

HEAD CIRCUMFERENCE—GIRLS

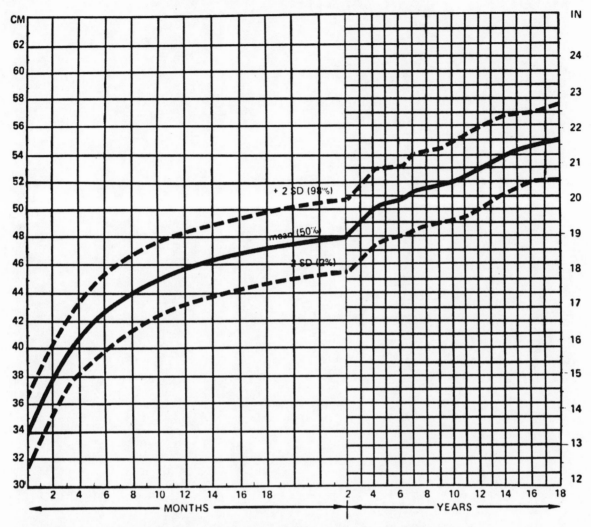

Ref: NELLHAUS, G., Composite International & Interracial Graphs, Pediatrics *41:*106, 1968

FORMS FOR IMMUNIZATIONS

IMMUNIZATION INFORMATION SHEETS

Immunizations are usually given by public health departments, but sometimes by the school nurse—rarely by an aide or LVN (LPN).

The paraprofessional, however, often has the responsibility of determining that a particular student is in full compliance with state law and that all the shots are up to date. For this, some inservice training is required.

The three forms are for those school (or public health) nurses who administer legally mandated immunization vaccines. These forms are furnished by the Center for Disease Control in Atlanta, Georgia, and may be obtained through local health departments.

NOTE: The three forms shown here are used by the San Antonio (Texas) Metropolitan Health District and are for illustration only. Be sure to use forms for your particular school district.

STATE LAW IMMUNIZATION REQUIREMENTS

The State Law Immunization Requirements should be furnished to the parents of any child who is not in compliance with state law regarding immunization and who are reluctant, for whatever reasons, to have their child receive the necessary immunizations.

The form must, of course, be adapted to meet individual state needs.

PROVISIONAL ENROLLMENT NOTICE

Since each state's immunization law varies in some detail, forms such as the Provisional Enrollment Notice must be modified to comply with that state's statutes as well as the school district's policy regarding allowing a student to enroll in school pending receipt of immunization record and/or completion of a series of immunizations that have begun.

The state immunization requirements for school attendance can always be obtained from the local, regional, or state health department office.

RELIGIOUS EXEMPTION FROM IMMUNIZATION

Religious and medical exemption from state immunization requirements are permitted. There are differences in the wording of the law from state to state, however, so that forms of this nature must be written to comply with the statute.

There are also some nonreligious objections to immunizations, such as the belief that introducing "foreign substances" into the body is unnatural. Such reasons are usually denied religious exemption from immunization.

The Religious Exemption from Immunization was written to comply with Texas law.

PRE-IMMUNIZATION QUESTIONNAIRE AND MEDICAL EXEMPTION

The "Pre-Immunization Questionnaire and Medical Exemption" is completed by the parent and/or physician to avoid untoward immunization reactions and provide valid medical exemptions when necessary. Most states allow non-immunized children to remain in school if there is a valid medical reason.

CLINIC WORKSHEET

The Clinic Worksheet is for school districts whose nurses give immunizations. It is a convenient worksheet to record shots given prior to entering the information on the student's permanent health record.

IMPORTANT INFORMATION ABOUT MEASLES, MUMPS, AND RUBELLA VACCINES

Instructions: **Please read this carefully.**

What is measles? Measles is the most serious of the common childhood diseases. Usually it causes a rash, high fever, cough, runny nose, and watery eyes lasting 1 to 2 weeks. Sometimes it is more serious. It causes an ear infection or pneumonia in nearly 1 out of 10 children who get it. Approximately 1 child out of every 1,000 who get measles has an inflammation of the brain (encephalitis). This can lead to convulsions, deafness, or mental retardation. About 2 children in every 10,000 who get measles die from it. Measles can also cause a pregnant woman to have a miscarriage or give birth to a premature baby.

Before measles vaccine shots were available, there were hundreds of thousands of cases and hundreds of deaths each year. Nearly all children got measles by the time they were 15. Now, wide use of measles vaccine has nearly eliminated measles from the United States. However, if children are not vaccinated, they have a high risk of getting measles, either now or later in life.

What is mumps? Mumps is a common disease of children. Usually it causes fever, headache, and inflammation of the salivary glands, which causes the cheeks to swell. Sometimes it is more serious. It causes inflammation of the coverings of the brain and spinal cord (meningitis) in about 1 child in every 10 who get it. More rarely, it can cause inflammation of the brain (encephalitis), which usually goes away without leaving permanent damage. Mumps can also cause deafness. About 1 out of every 4 adolescent or adult men who get mumps develops painful inflammation and swelling of the testicles. While this condition usually goes away, on rare occasions it may cause sterility.

Before mumps vaccine shots were available, there were more than 150,000 cases each year. Now, because of the wide use of mumps vaccine, the number of cases of mumps is much lower. However, if children are not vaccinated, they have a high risk of getting mumps.

What is rubella? Rubella is also called German measles. It is a common disease of children and may also affect adults. Usually it is very mild and causes a slight fever, rash, and swelling of glands in the neck. The sickness lasts about 3 days. Sometimes, especially in adult women, there may be swelling and aching of the joints for a week or two. Very rarely, rubella can cause inflammation of the brain (encephalitis) or cause a temporary bleeding disorder (purpura).

The most serious problem with rubella is that if a pregnant woman gets this disease, there is a good chance that she may have a miscarriage or that the baby will be born crippled, blind, or with other defects. The last big rubella epidemic in the United States was in 1964. Because of that epidemic, about 25,000 children were born with serious problems such as heart defects, deafness, blindness, or mental retardation because their mothers had rubella during the pregnancy.

Before rubella vaccine shots were available, rubella was so common that most children got the disease by the time they were 15. Now, because of the wide use of rubella vaccine, the number of cases of rubella is much lower. However, if children are not vaccinated, they have a high risk of getting rubella and possibly exposing a pregnant woman to the disease. If an unvaccinated woman later becomes pregnant and catches rubella, she may have a defective baby.

Since rubella is a mild illness, many women of childbearing age do not recall if they had rubella as a child. A simple blood test can show whether a person is immune to rubella or is not protected against the disease. Overall, about 1 in 5 women of childbearing age is not protected against rubella.

Measles, mumps, and rubella vaccines: The vaccines are given by injection and are very effective. Ninety percent or more of people who get the shot will have protection, probably for life. Since protection is not as likely to occur if the vaccines are given very early in life, these vaccines should be given to children after their first birthday; measles vaccine should be given at 15 months of age or older. Measles, mumps, and rubella vaccines can be given one at a time or in a combined vaccine (measles-rubella [MR], measles-mumps-rubella [MMR]) by a single shot. If they are given in combined vaccine, they should be given at 15 months of age or older.

Experts recommend that adolescents and adults—especially women of child-bearing age—who are not known to be immune to rubella should receive rubella vaccine (or MMR if they might also be susceptible to measles or mumps). Women should not receive the shot if they are pregnant or might become pregnant within 3 months. There is no known risk in being vaccinated against any or all three of these diseases if you are already immune to any of them.

Possible side effects from the vaccines: About 1 out of every 5 children will get a rash or slight fever lasting for a few days, 1 or 2 weeks after getting measles vaccine. Occasionally there is mild swelling of the salivary glands after mumps vaccination.

About 1 out of every 7 children who gets rubella vaccine will get a rash or some swelling of the glands of the neck 1 or 2 weeks after the shot. About 1 out of every 20 children who gets rubella vaccine will have some aching or swelling of the joints. This may happen anywhere from 1 to 3 weeks after the shot. It usually lasts only 2 or 3 days. Adults are more likely to have these problems with their joints—as many as 1 in 4 may have them. Other temporary side effects, such as pain, numbness, or tingling in the hands and feet have also occurred but are very uncommon.

Although experts are not sure, it seems that *very rarely* children who get these vaccines may have a more serious reaction, such as inflammation of the brain (encephalitis), convulsions with fever, or nerve deafness.

With any vaccine or drug, there is a possibility that allergic or other more serious reactions or even death could occur.

Warning—some persons should *not* take these vaccines without checking with a doctor:

- Anyone who is sick right now with something more serious than a cold.
- Anyone who had an allergic reaction to eating eggs so serious that it required medical treatment (does not apply to rubella vaccine).
- Anyone with cancer, leukemia, or lymphoma.
- Anyone with a disease that lowers the body's resistance to infection.
- Anyone taking a drug that lowers the body's resistance to infection (such as cortisone, prednisone, or certain anticancer drugs).
- Anyone who has received a gamma globulin (immune globulin) within the preceding 3 months.
- Anyone who had an allergic reaction to an antibiotic called neomycin so serious that it required medical treatment.

Pregnancy: Measles, mumps, and rubella vaccines are not known to cause special problems for pregnant women or their unborn babies. However, doctors usually avoid giving any drugs or vaccines to pregnant women unless there is a specific need. To be safe, pregnant women should not get these vaccines. A woman who gets any of these vaccines should wait 3 months before getting pregnant.

Vaccinating a child whose mother is pregnant is not dangerous to the pregnancy.

Questions: If you have any questions about measles, mumps, or rubella vaccination, please ask us now or call your doctor or health department before you sign this form.

Reactions: If the person who received the vaccine gets sick and visits a doctor, hospital, or clinic in the 4 weeks after vaccination, please report it to:

PLEASE KEEP THIS PART OF THE INFORMATION SHEET FOR YOUR RECORDS

I have read the information on this form about measles, mumps, and rubella vaccines. I have had a chance to ask questions that were answered to my satisfaction. I believe I understand the benefits and risks of measles, mumps, and rubella vaccines and request that the vaccine checked below be given to me or to the person named below for whom I am authorized to make this request.

VACCINE TO BE GIVEN: Measles _____ Mumps _____ Rubella _____ Measles-Rubella _____ Measles-Mumps-Rubella _____

INFORMATION ON PERSON TO RECEIVE VACCINE (Please print first four lines)					FOR CLINIC USE	
Name (last) (first) (middle)			Birthdate	Sex	Clinic code	Vaccine code
Address	Zip code		Telephone number		Date vaccinated	
					MSD	
City	State				Manufacturer and lot number	
Mother's name (last) (first) X					Site of administration	
					☐ New	☐ Repeat
Signature of person authorized to make the request			Date		Type record	

IMPORTANT INFORMATION ABOUT POLIO AND ORAL POLIO VACCINE

Instructions: Please read this carefully.

What is polio? Polio is a virus disease that may cause permanent crippling (paralysis) and occasionally death. There used to be thousands of cases and hundreds of deaths from polio every year in the United States. Because of the widespread use of polio vaccines, which became available beginning in the mid-1950s, polio disease has nearly been eliminated from the United States. Although thousands of cases continue to occur each year in the rest of the world, in the United States during the past 5 years there have been only 67 cases of polio reported, an average of 13 cases per year. Our success in preventing the spread of wild polio virus has been so great that most of the recent cases (approximately nine per year) have resulted from the rare side effects of oral polio vaccine (see below). Because of this fact, some people have asked why we should continue to use polio vaccine. The reason is that, even though we may not have much wild polio virus spreading here now, there is so much of it in the rest of the world that there is a great risk of its being reestablished if our children are not vaccinated.

Oral live polio vaccine: Immunization with oral live polio vaccine (OPV) is one of the best ways to prevent polio. It is given by mouth starting in early infancy. Several doses are needed to provide good protection. Young children should get two or more doses in the first year of life and another dose at about 18 months of age. An additional dose is important for children when they enter school or when there is a high risk of polio, for example, during an epidemic or when traveling to a place where polio is common. The vaccine is easy to take and is effective in preventing the spread of polio. In over 90 percent of people, OPV gives protection for a long time, probably for life. Because OPV viruses live for a time in the intestinal tract of the person who is vaccinated, some of the viruses pass in the stool and can spread from the vaccinated person to those in close contact (usually household members). This may help to immunize these persons and is one of the advantages of OPV. The Immunization Practices Advisory Committee of the Public Health Service and the American Academy of Pediatrics recommended oral live polio vaccine as the preferred polio vaccine for people up to the eighteenth birthday.

Possible side effects from the vaccine: OPV very rarely (once in about every 8.1 million doses of OPV distributed) causes paralytic polio in the person who is vaccinated. The risk may be slightly higher in adults being vaccinated and substantially higher in persons with abnormally low resistance to infection. Also very rarely (once in about every 5 million doses of OPV distributed) paralytic polio may develop in a close contact of a recently vaccinated person. Even though these risks are very low, they should be recognized. The risk of side effects from the vaccine must be balanced against the risk of the disease, both now and in the future.

Pregnancy: Polio vaccine experts do not think oral polio vaccine can cause special problems for pregnant women or their unborn babies. However, doctors usually avoid giving any drugs or vaccines to pregnant women unless there is a specific need. Pregnant women should check with a doctor before taking oral polio vaccine.

Warning—some persons should not take oral polio vaccine without checking with a doctor:

- Anyone with cancer, leukemia, or lymphoma.
- Anyone with a disease that lowers the body's resistance to infection.
- Anyone taking a drug that lowers the body's resistance to infection, such as cortisone or prednisone.
- Anyone who lives in the same household with anyone who has one of the conditions listed above.
- Anyone who is sick right now with something more serious than a cold.
- Pregnant women.
- Most persons age 18 and older because adults have a slightly bigger risk of developing paralysis from oral polio vaccine than children. (However, if the risk of polio is increased—as may occur, for example, when there is an outbreak in your community—most polio experts recommend that unprotected persons receive oral polio vaccine regardless of age.)

Note of injectable (killed) polio vaccine: Besides the oral polio vaccine (OPV), there is also a killed polio vaccine (IPV) given by injection which protects against polio after several shots. This killed polio vaccine has no known risk of causing paralytic polio. Because OPV may provide lifetime protection, seems to provide stronger immunity in the intestinal tract (where infection first occurs), is simpler to administer, and is more effective in preventing the spread of polio virus than IPV, most polio experts feel that oral vaccine is more effective for controlling polio in the United States. Injectable polio vaccine is recommended for persons needing polio vaccination who have low resistance to serious infections or who live with persons with low resistance to serious infections. It may also be recommended for previously unvaccinated adults who plan to travel to a place where polio is common or for previously unvaccinated adults whose children are to be vaccinated with OPV. It is not widely used in this country at the present time, but it is available. If you would like to know more about this type of polio vaccine, or wish to receive this vaccine, please ask us.

Questions: If you have any questions about polio or polio vaccination, please ask us now or call your doctor or health department before you sign this form.

Reactions: If the person who received the vaccine gets sick and visits a doctor, hospital, or clinic in the 4 weeks after vaccination, please report it to:

PLEASE KEEP THIS PART OF THE INFORMATION SHEET FOR YOUR RECORDS

I have read the information on this form about polio and the oral vaccine. I have had a chance to ask questions that were answered to my satisfaction. I believe I understand the benefits and risks of oral polio vaccine and request that it be given to me or to the person named below for whom I am authorized to make this request.

INFORMATION ON PERSON TO RECEIVE VACCINE (Please print first four lines)						FOR CLINIC USE	
							OPV
Name (last)	(first)		(middle)	Birthdate	Sex	Clinic code	Vaccine code
Address		Zip code		Telephone number		Date vaccinated	
						LED	
City		State				Manufacturer and lot number	
						ORAL	
Mother's name (last)				(first)		Site of administration	
X						☐ New	☐ Repeat
Signature of person authorized to make the request				Date		Type record	

132

IMPORTANT INFORMATION ABOUT DIPHTHERIA, TETANUS, AND PERTUSSIS AND DTP, DT, AND Td VACCINES

Instructions: Please read this carefully.

What is diphtheria? Diphtheria is a very serious disease that can affect people in different ways. It can cause an infection in the nose and throat that can interfere with breathing. It can also cause an infection of the skin. Sometimes it causes heart failure or paralysis. About 1 person out of every 10 who gets diphtheria dies of it.

What is tetanus? Tetanus, or lockjaw, results when wounds are infected with tetanus bacteria, which are often found in dirt. The bacteria in the wound make a poison which causes the muscles of the body to go into spasm. Four out of every 10 persons who get tetanus die of it.

What is pertussis? Pertussis, or whooping cough, causes severe spells of coughing that can interfere with eating, drinking, and breathing. In the United States, more than 75 percent of reported pertussis cases occur in children younger than 5 years. Pertussis is a more serious disease in young children and more than half of the children reported to have pertussis are hospitalized. In recent years, an average of 1,700 cases of pertussis have been reported each year in the United States. Complications occur in a substantial proportion of reported cases. Pneumonia occurs in 1 of every 4 children with pertussis. For every 1,000 reported pertussis cases, 40 develop convulsions and 4 develop inflammation of the brain. In recent years, an average of nine deaths due to pertussis occurred each year.

Before vaccines were developed, these three diseases were all very common and caused a large number of deaths each year in the United States. If children are not vaccinated, the risk of getting these diseases will go back up again.

DTP, DT, and Td vaccines: Immunization with DTP vaccine is one of the best ways to prevent these diseases. DTP vaccine is actually three vaccines combined into one shot to make it easier to get protection. The vaccine is given by injection starting early in infancy. Several shots are needed to get good protection. Young children should get three doses in the first year of life and a fourth dose at about 18 months of age. A booster shot is important for children who are about to enter school, and should be given between their fourth and seventh birthdays. The vaccine is very effective at preventing tetanus—over 95 percent of those who get the vaccine are protected if the recommended number of shots is given. Although the diphtheria and pertussis parts of the vaccine are not quite as effective, they still prevent most children from getting a disease and they make the disease milder for those who do get it.

Because pertussis is not very common or severe in older children, those 7 years of age and older should take a vaccine that does not contain the pertussis part. Also, because reactions to the diphtheria part of the vaccine may be more common in older children, those 7 years of age and older should take a form of the vaccine that has a lower concentration of the diphtheria part. This vaccine that contains no pertussis part and a lower concentration of the diphtheria part is called Td vaccine. Boosters with the Td vaccine should be received every 10 years throughout life.

Deferral of DTP Immunization: Some children who are less than 7 years of age and have had a serious reaction to previous DTP shots should not receive additional pertussis vaccine. A preparation called DT vaccine is available for them that does not contain the pertussis part. Also, children who have previously had a convulsion should generally not receive DTP vaccine until it can be determined that an evolving neurological disorder is not present.

The United States Public Health Service and the American Academy of Pediatrics recommended DTP vaccine be used in children up to 7 years of age unless they have had a serious reaction to earlier shots or have a neurologic disorder.

Possible side effects from the vaccine: With DTP vaccine, most children will have a slight fever and be irritable within 2 days after getting the shot. One-half of children develop some soreness and swelling in the area where the shot was given. More serious side effects can occur. A temperature greater than 102° F may follow 1 out of 20 DTP shots. Convulsions or episodes of limpness and paleness may each occur after 1 in every 1,750 shots. Children who have previously had a convulsion may be more likely to have another one after pertussis shots. Unusual, high-pitched crying may occur after 1 in every 1,000 shots. Rarely, about once in every 110,000 shots, inflammation of the brain (encephalitis) may occur and permanent brain damage may occur about once in every 310,000 shots. Side effects from DT or Td vaccine are not common and usually consist only of soreness and slight fever.

Warning—some persons should *not* take these vaccines without checking with a doctor:
- Anyone who is sick right now with something more serious than a cold.
- Anyone who has had a convulsion or other problems of the nervous system.
- Anyone who has had a serious reaction to DTP shots before, such as a temperature of 105° F or greater, a convulsion, an episode of limpness and paleness, unusual high-pitched crying, or inflammation of the brain (encephalitis).

Questions: If you have any questions about diphtheria, tetanus, or pertussis or DTP, DT, or Td vaccination, please ask us now or call your doctor or health department before you sign this form.

Reactions: If the person who received the vaccine gets sick and visits a doctor, hospital, or clinic in the 4 weeks after vaccination, please report it to:

PLEASE KEEP THIS PART OF THE INFORMATION SHEET FOR YOUR RECORDS

I have read the information on this form about diphtheria, tetanus, and pertussis and DTP, DT, and Td vaccines. I have had a chance to ask questions that were answered to my satisfaction. I believe I understand the benefits and risks of DTP, DT, and Td vaccines and request that the vaccine checked below be given to me or to the person named below for whom I am authorized to make this request. VACCINE TO BE GIVEN: DTP _____ DT _____ Td _____

INFORMATION ON PERSON TO RECEIVE VACCINE (Please print first four lines)						FOR CLINIC USE	
						Clinic code	Vaccine code
Name (last)	(first)	(middle)		Birthdate	Sex	Date vaccinated	
Address	Zip code			Telephone number		Manufacturer and lot number	
City	State					Site of administration	
Mother's name (last)		(first)					
X						☐ New	☐ Repeat
Signature of person authorized to make the request				Date		Type record	

133

PARENTAL NOTIFICATION FOLLOWING IMMUNIZATION

Immunizations as indicated below were given to _____
                                                     Student's name

Date of birth _____ **School no.** _____ **I.D. no.** _____

Diphtheria-Pertussis-Tetanus

Injection 1 _____	
	Date
Injection 2 _____	
	Date
Injection 3 _____	
	Date
Booster _____	
	Date

Diphtheria-Tetanus

Injection 1 _____
                     Date

Injection 2 _____
                     Date

Booster _____
                 Date

Oral Polio

Injection 1 _____
                     Date

Injection 2 _____
                     Date

Booster _____
                 Date

Mumps

Injection _____
                   Date

Measles-Mumps-Rubella

Injection _____
                     Date

Rubeola

Injection _____
                     Date

Rubella

Injection _____
                     Date

Please keep this information for your health records.

_____
School nurse

134

IMMUNIZATION AND SCREENING DATA

Instructions: Record all immunizations.

Name (full) _____ **Birthdate** _____ **Grade** _____

Address _____ **Telephone** _____

Parent or guardian _____

DPT or Td _____ _____ _____ _____ _____ _____ _____
        Date 1   Date 2   Date 3   Date 4   Date 5   Date 6   Physician

Oral polio _____ _____ _____ _____ _____ _____ _____
        Date 1   Date 2   Date 3   Date 4   Date 5   Date 6   Physician

Rubeola _____ _____ _____
        Date of vaccine   Date of disease   Physician

Rubella _____   _____
        Date of vaccine   Physician

Mumps _____ _____ _____
        Date of vaccine   Date of disease   Physician

Vision   R _____   L _____   Date of test _____

Hearing   R _____   L _____   Date of test _____

Schools are reminded that transfer of immunization records is required by law (in some states).

REQUEST FOR IMMUNIZATION RECORDS
(English)

Our records indicate that your child, _____,
does not have up-to-date immunizations as required by state law.

According to our records your child needs

Diphtheria–pertussis–tetanus (DPT) _____   Measles _____

Tetanus–diphtheria (TD) _____   Mumps _____

Polio _____   Rubella _____

If your child has received the shots, please send the records to school so that his or her health card may be updated. Your records will be returned immediately.

If your child has not received the shots, please take him or her to your family doctor or to a public health clinic to receive the shots. If you wish the school nurse to give the shots, please read and sign the attached form/forms and return them to the nurse.

_____   _____
Date   School nurse

_____
School

Departamento de Salubridad

Requisito de Documentos de Vacunas
(Spanish)

Nuestros documentos indican que su niño/niña no ha recibido las vacunas que la ley de requiere.

Su niño/niña necesita recibir las vacunas que se han marcado.

Difteria, tétano, tosferina _____   Paperas (Chanza) _____

Tétano y difteria _____   Sarampión (Rubeola) _____

Polio _____   Sarampión aleman _____

Si su niño/niña tiene las vacunas necesarias por favor mande sus documentos oficiales que notan la fecha y clase de vacuna que ha recibido. Sus documentos seran regresados enseguida.

Si su niño/niña no ha recibido las vacunas necesarias por favor llevelo con su médico o clinica de salud. Y si gusta firme los permisos necesarios y la enfermera dará las vacunas indicadas.

_____   _____
Fecha   Enfermera

_____
Escuela

ADDITIONAL IMMUNIZATION/INFORMATION NEEDED

Pupil's name		D.O.B.	School		Grade	Date

Dear Parent:

According to our school records, your child needs additional immunizations or additional information regarding the dates that the immunizations were given to meet the Health and Safety Code requirements to remain enrolled in school. The immunizations may be obtained from your family physician or at no cost from the County Health Department. During the school year immunizations are available at no extra cost at the Unified School District Clinic.

For Polio, DPT, and TD, the *last dose* must be *after* the second birthday and at least 6 months must have elapsed between the last 2 doses.

The records indicate the student needs the immunization circled:

Polio:	1	2	3	4	5
DPT:	1	2	3	4	5
TD:	1	2	3	4	

The records indicate that we do not have the month and year that circled vaccine was given

Polio:	1	2	3	4	5
DPT:	1	2	3	4	5
TD:	1	2	3	4	

Immunization for measles, mumps, and rubella must be given *after* the first birthday; therefore the *day* as well as the month and year must be recorded if given in the same month as child's birthday.

Measles:	1	2
Mumps:	1	2
Rubella:	1	2

Measles: _____
Month-day-year given

Mumps: _____
Month-day-year given

Rubella: _____
Month-day-year given

If you have lost your records and specific immunization dates are not available, the law states that you may enter the month and year of each polio, DPT, and TD or the month, day, and year of measles, mumps, and rubella vaccine to the *best of your recollection.* Your signature on the form is required if you are providing dates and means that you assume all liability for the protection of your child from the diseases listed above.

You must send to school the dates requested or verification that your child has received the vaccine circled above by _____.
Date

Failure to comply will result in

_____ Your child being excluded from school on _____.

_____ Your child will not be allowed to enroll in junior or senior high school until verification of immunization and/or required dates have been received by the school.

We sincerely thank you for your cooperation in protecting the health of students.

_____
Signature of parent/guardian   Date

137

SCHOOL HEALTH SERVICES PARENTAL LETTER
(English)

To the parents of _____

Date _____

Dear Parent:

Our records indicate that _____ _____ _____
I.D. Grade/Section

needs immunization described below on or before _____ **in order to attend school.**
Date

When your child has completed the immunizations, please submit the official record of immunization to the nurse or school principal. Immunizations may be obtained from your private physician or a neighborhood public health center. If your child has known allergies or is under treatment for an acute illness or a chronic health problem, the immunizations may be given only through your physician's office.

The parent or legal guardian must accompany the student to the clinic. In the event that a parent escort is not possible, the school nurse or public health clinic should be contacted for specific information related to signed parent permission for immunization.

Your school nurse

_____
School

_____
Principal

To the physician

<table>
<tr><td colspan="4">

Our records indicate that this student has had the following immunizations:

	Dose 1	Dose 2	Booster
Dip/Tet	_____	_____	_____
Polio	_____	_____	_____
Measles (rubeola)	_____	_____	_____
Rubella	_____	_____	_____
Mumps	_____	_____	_____

☐ We have no record of immunization.

</td><td colspan="4">

To comply with state guidelines, this student needs the following immunizations:

	Dosage due	Date administered	Physician/ clinic
Dip/Tet	_____	_____	_____
Polio	_____	_____	_____
Measles (rubeola)	_____	_____	_____
Rubella	_____	_____	_____
Mumps	_____	_____	_____

</td></tr>
</table>

If protected by disease (measles/mumps) initial the following statement:
The above-named student had (measles/mumps) illness on date specified above and does not need related immunization. _____
Initial here

Verification of updates above: _____ _____
Physician's signature   Telephone

138

SCHOOL HEALTH SERVICES PARENTAL LETTER
(Spanish)

Fecha _____

A los Padres de _____

Estimados Padres:

Nuestros archivos nos indican que _____

necesita que se le apliquen las vacunas que se describen en seguida antes del _____
FECHA (Compliance Data)

para poder asistir a la escuela.

Cuando su hijo/hija haya completado su dosis de inmunización, haga favor de presentar el registro oficial de vacunas a la enfermera o al director de la escuela. Las vacunas las pueden obtener con su médico particular o a través de un centro público de salud en su vecindario. Si su hijo/hija tiene alguna alergia, o está bajo tratamiento a causa de una enfermedad aguda, o de algún problema crónico de salud, las vacunas sólo podrán ser obtenidas a través de su médico particular.

Los padres o el tutor, deben acompañar al estudiante a la clinica. En caso de que los padres no puedan acompañar al estudiante, les rogamos que se pongan en contacto con la enfermera de la escuela o con la clínica pública de salud, para que reciban la información relacionada con la firma de una carta por medico de la cuál autoricen a su hijo/hija a recibir la inmunización necesaria.

_____   **La enfermera de la escuela**
School

_____
Principal

To the physician

Our records indicate that this student has had the following immunizations:			
	Dose 1	Dose 2	Booster
Dip/Tet	_____	_____	_____
Polio	_____	_____	_____
Measles (rubeola)	_____	_____	_____
Rubella	_____	_____	_____
Mumps	_____	_____	_____
☐ We have no record of immunization.			

To comply with state guidelines, this student needs the following immunizations:		
	Dosage due	Date administered	Physician/clinic
Dip/Tet	_____	_____	_____
Polio	_____	_____	_____
Measles (rubeola)	_____	_____	_____
Rubella	_____	_____	_____
Mumps	_____	_____	_____

If protected by disease (measles/mumps), initial the following statement:
The above-named student had (measles/mumps) illness on date specified above and does not need related immunization. _____
Initial here

Verification of updates above: _____   _____
Physician's signature   Telephone

139

STATE LAW IMMUNIZATION REQUIREMENTS

Dear Parent or guardian:

Our files indicate that your child, _____, does not have up-to-date immunization records as required by state law. The school nurse has made the following attempts to obtain this information:

_____

_____

_____

The law directs us not to allow students with incomplete immunization records to attend school. Therefore, your child may not attend school after _____ unless the records are completed.

A certificate signed by a physician licensed to practice in the United States or officially stamped by a recognized health agency (example: city or state health department) with dates of immunizations indicated must be presented to the school immediately. If your child has received immunizations recently and the school has not seen the records, please send the records to school. The requirements are as follow:

1. DTP (diphtheria-tetanus-whooping cough)—up to the sixth birthdate minimum of three doses, one dose since fourth birthdate.

2. DT (diphtheria-tetanus)—after the sixth birthdate. Minimum of three doses, one dose since fourth birthdate and last dose within the past ten years.

3. Polio—minimum of three doses, last dose since fourth birthdate (oral polio vaccine).

4. Measles—one dose after first birthdate or actual illness and after January 1, 1968.

5. Rubella—one dose (history of actual illness not acceptable).

6. Mumps—one dose or actual illness.

If your child has actually had red measles or mumps, the immunization shot is not required, but a written history of having had the disease must be signed by a physician licensed to practice in the United States.

_____
Principal

According to our records your child needs

_____ _____ _____ _____

_____ _____ _____ _____

_____ _____ _____ _____

_____ _____ _____ _____

STATE LAW MINIMUM IMMUNIZATION REQUIREMENTS FOR SCHOOL ATTENDANCE SCHOOL YEAR 19__

Up to Sixth Birthdate

Vaccine	No. of doses	Remarks
DTP	3	One dose must have been given after fourth birthdate.
Oral polio	3	One dose must have been given after fourth birthdate.
Measles	1	Must be after first birthdate.
Rubella	1	
Mumps	1	

After Sixth Birthdate

TD	3	One dose must have been given after fourth birthdate and the last dose within ten years.
Oral polio	3	One dose must have been given after fourth birthdate.
Measles	1	Required of all students after first birthdate—must have been given after January 1, 1968.
Rubella	1	Not required after twelfth birthdate.
Mumps	1	Required up to the ____ birthdate (increase one year of age each September 1).

IMMUNIZATION ASSESSMENT

The school nurse or designated school personnel will ensure that all students enrolled are in compliance with the state immunization laws.

Rationale

To minimize the number of preventable communicable diseases, the legislature has enacted laws regarding the immunizations required for school attendance. All pupils enrolled in any public or private school throughout the state must meet these requirements. The nurse is the appropriate person to review, evaluate, and oversee compliance of the immunization statutes.

Structure Criteria

1. The state immunization requirements are as follows:

All students entering any new school K–12			In addition
Trivalent polio I.V.P. and/or any combination	3 doses 4 doses	One more dose if last dose before second birthdate.	**Ninth Grade** Until February 1985, the records of all ninth-grade students must be reviewed to assure that rubella requirements are met.
DTP and/or any combination Td or DT	4 doses 3 doses	One more dose if last dose before second birthdate.	**Seventh Grade** Until February 1987, the records of all seventh-grade students must be reviewed to assure that rubella requirements are met.
Measles vaccine	1 dose	One more dose if given before first birthdate or before 1968.	**Measles disease or vaccine before 1968** Must be verified by doctor. Vaccine must have been a live virus vaccine and include date and type of vaccine.
Rubella Twelfth graders, except those from out of state, are exempt during 1984–1985	1 dose	One more dose if given before first birthdate or before June 1969.	**Rubella and mumps disease** Must be laboratory confirmed and verified in writing.
Mumps Required only to seventh birthdate	1 dose	One more dose if given before first birthdate.	**Below kindergarten age** Use age-appropriate immunization schedule.

2. The law provides for *conditional* admission when immunizations have been given appropriately, and the pupil is in a waiting period for the next required dose.

3. Exemption from the immunization requirements are limited by law to the specific circumstances listed below:

> *Contrary to personal beliefs:* Requires that parent/guardian sign a written statement that immunizations are contrary to their personal beliefs.
>
> *Medical contraindication:* Requires a *written* statement by a physician that specifies the reason for medical exemption, the immunizations that are contraindicated, and the probable duration of the exemption.

142

PROVISIONAL ENROLLMENT NOTICE

To the parent or guardian of _____

D.O.B. _____

        Although this child has not been fully immunized according to state law, he or she is being granted provisional or temporary enrollment for the following reason:

☐ Immunizations have begun, but are not completed. Completion of state-mandated immunizations must be given as rapidly as medically feasible.

☐ Student has transferred from another school and the immunization record is being transferred. Record must be received within 30 days.

        Consult your school nurse for further information.

Date _____ School _____ Principal _____

        A copy of this document will be kept by the school nurse who will maintain and monitor adequate immunization records.

NOTICE OF EXCLUSION FROM SCHOOL EFFECTIVE _____

Dear Parent or guardian:

State law requires all students attending grades 7 through 10 to have satisfactory evidence on file at school of having received live measles and rubella vaccines on or after the first birthday. For students in grades 11 and 12, measles vaccine is required and rubella vaccine is highly recommended. A recent review of our school records found_____'s record to be unsatisfactory for the reason(s) circled below:

Code	Measles	Rubella	Reason
A	_____	_____	No record is on file.
B	_____	_____	Immunization received before the first birthday and must be repeated.
C	_____	_____	Incomplete date of immunization. At least the month and year received are required.
D	_____	_____	No date of immunization, just a checkmark in the school record. At least month and year received are required.
E	_____	_____	Immunization received during the month of the first birthday. Day of immunization is needed to document that it was on or after the first birthday.
F	_____	_____	History of disease, no immunization received: physician verification is required for measles. Laboratory evidence of immunity is required for rubella.
G	_____	_____	Measles immunization of an unknown type received prior to 1968 or rubella vaccine received prior to June 1969, its date of licensure in the United States.

Other

_____ _____ _____ _____

The parent or guardian must submit to this school a record that documents that the above-named student has received live measles and rubella vaccine on or after the first birthday. The record must include at least the month and year received. Students will not be admitted after the *exclusion* date unless the immunization requirements have been met. Should you have any questions or require additional information, please call _____.

Thank you for your prompt attention to this matter.

Sincerely,

Principal

ENGLISH/SPANISH TRANSLATION OF IMMUNIZATIONS TERMS

English

1. Smallpox
2. Polio
3. BCG
4. DTP (diphtheria, tetanus, pertussis)
5. Rubeola
6. Tetanus
7. Typhoid
8. TB test (Mantoux)
9. Rubella (German measles)
10. Mumps

Spanish

Antivariolosa or viruela
Antipolio
BCG
DTP (Difteria, tétanos, tosferina)
Sarampión
Tetanos
Antitifoidica or antitifoidea
Tuberculinica (Mantoux)
Rubela (sarampión aleman)
Paperas ó parotitis

RELIGIOUS EXEMPTION FROM IMMUNIZATION

I hereby affirm that

   1. I am a member of the

   _____
   Name of church

   and

   2. Immunization as required by state law for school attendance conflicts with the tenets and practices of my religion.

Name of student _____

Name of parent or guardian _____

Address _____ **Phone** _____

_____   _____
Date   **Signature of parent or guardian**

_____

I am an ordained minister of the above-named church, a recognized religious organization, and have access to the membership records. The above-named person is a bona fide member of the church. Immunization of said child would be contrary to the tenets and practices of the

   _____
   Name of church

Name _____

Address _____ **Phone** _____

_____   _____
Date   **Signature of minister**

The student must present an affidavit signed by the applicant or, if a minor, by his or her parent or guardian stating that the immunization conflicts with the tenets and practices of a recognized church or religious denomination of which the applicant is an adherent or member provided, however, that this exemption does not apply in times of emergency or epidemic declared by the Commissioner of Health.

PREIMMUNIZATION QUESTIONNAIRE AND MEDICAL EXEMPTION

Name_____D.O.B._____Grade_____School_____

1. **My child is allergic to**
   Eggs? _____ Yes _____ No Neomycin? _____ Yes _____ No
   Other (specify): _____

2. **My child is currently receiving medication prescribed by a physician:** _____ Yes _____ No
   Medication (if any): _____

3. **My child had a reaction to an immunization?** _____ Yes _____ No
   If yes, specify: _____

4. **If girl, has begun to menstruate:** _____ Yes _____ No

5. **Has child had any immunizations in the past 30 days?** _____ Yes _____ No If yes, specify: _____

6. **My child must be exempted from the legally mandated immunizations for the following medical reasons.**

_____

_____

_____

_____

_____

_____ _____ _____
Parent's printed name   **Parent's signature**   **Phone**

_____ _____
Physician's printed name   **Physician's signature**

_____ _____ _____
Phone   **State lic. no.**   **Date**

CLINIC WORKSHEET

School: _____

Student's name/ birthdate	Age	Advisory or teacher	P.S.										
			P.R.										
			DPT	DT	Polio	MMR	Rubeola	Rubella	Mumps				
			1. 2. 3. B.	1. 2. B.	1. 2. 3. B.								
			1. 2. 3. B.	1. 2. B.	1. 2. 3. B.								
			1. 2. 3. B.	1. 2. B.	1. 2. 3. B.								
			1. 2. 3. B.	1. 2. B.	1. 2. 3. B.								
			1. 2. 3. B.	1. 2. B.	1. 2. 3. B.								
			1. 2. 3. B.	1. 2. B.	1. 2. 3. B.								
			1. 2. 3. B.	1. 2. B.	1. 2. 3. B.								
			1. 2. 3. B.	1. 2. B.	1. 2. 3. B.								
			1. 2. 3. B.	1. 2. B.	1. 2. 3. B.								

P.S., permission sent; P.R., permission received.

QUESTIONS FOR FEMALES 12 YEARS OF AGE AND OVER BEFORE ADMINISTERING RUBELLA VACCINE

1. **"Do you have menstrual periods?"**

   If no, give explanation, get signature and vaccinate.

2. **"When did you start?"**

3. **"When was your last period?"**

   If three weeks or less, give explanation at right, get signature and vaccinate.

If answer is more than three weeks, ask how frequently she menstruates or what her cycle is. If her period is *not* late:

   Give explanation at right, get signature and vaccinate.

If her period is late, tell her to come back when she has a period.

_____
Nurse's signature

_____
Student's signature

Explanation

Explain to female that she must not get pregnant for three months. "We do not know of anyone's baby being affected by rubella vaccine given to the mother before birth, but we do not want to take any chances, and we want you to know that it's important that you not get pregnant for three months."

Do you understand this explanation?

_____ Yes _____ No

Do you have any more questions?

_____

_____

_____

_____
Date

FORMS FOR MEDICATION

PERMISSION TO GIVE MEDICATION AT SCHOOL

Each state has specific laws governing the administration of medication at school. Some states require only that the medication be in the original prescription bottle, plus signed parental permission. Others require a specific school form be filled out and signed by the physician, a requirement that may cause delay in the child's receiving important medication.

The Permission to Give Medication at School is an important, frequently used form. Note that it requires a physician's signature for long-term medication, but it does not specify how soon after the parent brings the medicine to school the form must be returned to the principal. This allows the principal and school nurse to exercise judgment and not permit critical medication doses to be missed.

If state law or district policy requires the form be filled out and signed by a physician, school authorities have no option but to comply.

NOTE

When nonprofessionals give medication at school, it is wise for a registered school nurse to give the first one or two doses. Adverse medication reactions may occur after any dose, but if a severe reaction is going to occur, it is likely to be after the first or second dose.

It is not safe for children to bring their own medication to school. This should be done by a parent or responsible adult. School authorities should be extra cautious about permitting children to take their own medicine home with them; if anything happens (such as another child taking a dose and having an adverse reaction), the school is in legal jeopardy.

LONG-TERM MEDICATION-REPORTING FORM

The Long-Term Medication Reporting Form is used by the campus nurse, teacher, counselor, or principal for these two reasons:

1. To ensure that adverse medication reactions are reported.
2. To report student behavior before and during medication or other therapy.

The form is sent to the health office or private physician when

1. Ordered by district health office or personal physician.
2. There is a change in dose and/or schedule or the medication is discontinued.
3. There is an adverse reaction.
4. Student transfers or withdraws.

Children with epilepsy, attention deficiency disorder, conduct or other emotional disorders, Tourette's syndrome, or other similar conditions often take daily medications that frequently cause adverse side effects. A list of such adverse reactions, submitted in writing, assures school personnel of a record that the reaction was properly reported.

The Conners' scale at the bottom of the form is a widely used and simple format that was designed to identify hyperactive children. Each check is given a numerical score corresponding to the column it is in. A total of 15 to 20 is questionably diagnostic of hyperactivity, and a score over 20, while not positively diagnostic, is highly suggestive of hyperactivity. Also, a dramatic reduction in the total score is often seen when a hyperactive child is scored after a favorable response to medication or other form of therapy.

SUMMARIES

The summaries are specialized forms useful in large school districts with large numbers of children on psychoactive medication. There is a tendency for a school district to increase its reliance slowly on drug therapy for behavioral problems, thus neglecting behavior modification and educational methods of management. Annual collection of data on children receiving psychoactive medication alerts the professional school nurse and other personnel if the percentage of children receiving such medication goes up every year.

An annual report is necessary to determine if the children receiving the medication are indeed improving.

The following glossary explains the initials and words:

1. ADD—attention deficit disorder
2. W/O—without

3. W—with

4. Pervasive disorder—present terminology for conditions such as autism, childhood schizophrenia, and related disorders

5. Affective/anxiety disorder—present terminology for "mood" disorders such as depression, separation anxiety, school phobia, and related disorders

If these two forms are to be used by a health clerk or aide, supervision by a health professional is advisable.

CONSENT STATEMENT

The consent statement is designed specifically for parents of children who receive amphetamines for ADD. The purpose of the form is to inform parents fully of possible side effects of medication and for legal protection.

Different information is required for different medications, so each prescribing physician should provide an appropriate form for commonly used medications that are given at school. Examples are medications for epilepsy, asthma, and emotional disorders.

DAILY LOG OF MEDICATION ADMINISTRATION

The Daily Log of Medication Administration maintains a written record of each dose given.

The proper box is initialed *at the time* the medicine is given. This is standard procedure at hospitals and other health care facilities and should also be done at schools.

The form should be posted in a location easily accessible *to the person giving the medication.* If different individuals give a medication to the same child on different days, use a separate form—each easily accessible to the person giving the medication.

MEDICATION ENVELOPE

Place the following Medication Envelope sheet on a manila envelope in which medication is kept for each child.

REQUEST FORM FOR _____ MEDICATION

The Request form for _____ Medication is used if the district central health office maintains a formulary of medications. State pharmacy guidelines must be followed.

Usually a registered pharmacist acts as a consultant to the school district. If any of the medications in the clinic require a physician's prescription, it is necessary for the district to have a consultant physician also.

PERMISSION TO GIVE MEDICATION AT SCHOOL

Note to parents/guardians:

The _____ School District requires that all students who need medication during school hours must do the following:

1. Present a written consent form signed by the parent or legal guardian.
2. Bring the medication in the original prescription bottle, properly labeled by a registered pharmacist as prescribed by law.

Long-term medication (longer than 4 weeks) may be given by district personnel provided that the prescribing physician completes the district medication permission request form.

Name of student _____

Date of birth _____   School _____

To Be Completed by Physician

Name of medication _____

Size of tablet (in mg) _____ or, if liquid (mg/tsp) _____

Specific time(s) and dose(s) to be given at school _____

at home _____

Length of time _____

Are there any restrictions? _____   _____ If yes, what and how long?
 Yes   No

_____

_____   _____   _____
Printed name of physician   Signature of physician   Date

To Be Completed by Parent

I, _____, give permission for my child to receive the above medication as directed.

_____   _____
Date   Parent's/guardian's signature

                                                         _____
                                                         Telephone no.

PHYSICIAN STATEMENT

Under the provision of _____ when it is found necessary to place a child on medication during the school day, the school must have the following information:

Child's name _____

Diagnosis is _____

Dosage _____

Time schedule _____

Medication to be taken from _____ to _____.
                              Date   Date

_____
Doctor's signature

A note from the doctor, containing the foregoing information, will be acceptable.

155

PARENT'S REQUEST FOR GIVING MEDICINE AT SCHOOL

I request the school to see that my child _____

Grade _____ Teacher _____ receive prescribed

_____ by Doctor _____
      Name of medication

Pharmacy _____ Prescription number _____

Diagnosis _____ .

Dosage _____ Time _____

Beginning _____ to _____
           Date   Date

The medication should be delivered to the school nurse, principal, and/or the designee. It should be in a container properly labeled (pharmacy label) with the student's name, the physician's name, date of original prescription, and name of medicine.

A written statement from the prescribing physician detailing the administering of medication must accompany this request.

We, the parent, authorize the school to assist our child in taking oral medication and agree that we will not hold liable any member of the school staff or an individual of official capacity who is directed by us (the parents) and the school administrator to assist our child in taking said oral medication.

_____
Signature of parent or guardian

Date _____

156

MEDICATION TO BE GIVEN AT SCHOOL: SIGNED APPROVAL

Student _____ Age _____ D.O.B. _____
      Last name   **First**   **Middle**

School _____ Grade _____

Name and dose of medication	Form: (tab, cap, pill, other):	Number to be taken	Approximate time of day	Observed or assisted by (name, position)

Parents

Do you wish this child to receive medication at school? Yes _____ No _____

Please bring medication to the school (do not send with student). How often will medication be brought to school? Daily _____ Weekly _____ Other _____

The law allows any person (not necessarily a nurse) to assist in carrying out a physician's recommendations, and the school recognizes the desirability of responding to the physician's request. This accommodation on the part of the school is not legally required. Therefore, the persons signing this form are agreeing to hold the school and its personnel *free* from any or all suits that might arise from these arrangements.

_____
Signature of *both* parents (or guardians) if living with student   Address

Phone _____ Date _____

_____

Physician

Diagnosis or indication for medication _____

Precautions, if any _____

I would like to have a followup report, by phone, with the Nurse _____ Teacher _____ Principal _____ Psychologist _____ At the following intervals: Weekly _____ Monthly _____ Quarterly _____

Please discontinue this request as of this date: _____.
(After this date, a new form must be completed for changes or new orders.)

           M.D.
_____ _____ _____ _____ _____
Signature of physician   License #   Address   Phone   Date

LONG-TERM MEDICATION REPORTING FORM

To be completed by _____

Date of report _____

Name _____ **Birthdate** _____ **School** _____ **Grade** _____

Medication and dosage _____ **Diagnosis** _____

	Dose	**Dose**	**Dose**

Dose schedule   A.M.: **Home**   **Noon: Home**   P.M.: **Home**
(all prescribed doses)   **School** ☐   **School** ☐   **School** ☐
(Circle "Home" or "School.")   (Place √ in each box in which a dose is given.)

Date began initially _____ **Physician** _____

Date began this school year _____

Adverse effects of medication: ☐ **None**   ☐ **Drowsiness**   ☐ **Headache**
☐ **Loss of weight**   ☐ **Weight gain**   ☐ **Upset stomach**   ☐ **Loss of appetite**
☐ **Condition worse**   ☐ **Other (explain)** _____

Instructions: Place a √ in box that describes reaction. If reaction not listed, describe at "Other."

Additional comments:

_____
School nurse

Conners' Abbreviated Behavior Rating Scale

Instructions: Place a √ in each square that applies. Total each column and add the totals for a final score. (Score value of each check.)

	Not at all 0	Just a little 1	Pretty much 2	Very much 3
1. Restless or overactive, excitable, impulsive				
2. Disturbing to other children				
3. Failure to finish things started				
4. Short attention span				
5. Constant fidgeting				
6. Inattentive, easily distracted				
7. Demands must be met immediately				
8. Cries often and easily				
9. Mood changes quickly and drastically				
10. Temper outbursts, explosive and unpredictable behavior				
Total score of columns	_____	_____	_____	_____

_____
Signature classroom teacher

ANNUAL SUMMARY OF DRUG THERAPY WORKSHEET

School year _____

Name/school	Date of birth (age in years)	Medication name/dosage	Diagnosis ADD with hyp. ADD w/o hyp. Pervas. dis. Aff./anx. dis. Conduct dis.	Results Improved (mild, mod., marked) Worsened (mild, mod., severe) No change Inadequate follow-up	Comments and Follow-up

Nurse practitioner _____

PSYCHOACTIVE MEDICATION—ANNUAL STATISTICAL SUMMARY

Year _____

Results of Treatment

	No.	Improved	Worsened	No change	Inadequate follow-up	Male/Female
ADD with hyperactivity						
ADD without hyperactivity						
Pervasive disorder						
Affective/anxiety disorder						
Conduct disorder						
					Totals	

Age Distribution

Ages	3–5	6–8	9–12	13–18
ADD with hyperactivity				
ADD w/o hyperactivity				
Pervasive disorder				
Affective/anxiety disorder				
Conduct disorder				

Medications Used

Ritalin _____   Mellaril _____   Others (list):

Cylert _____   Tofranil _____   _____

Dexedrine _____   Stelazine _____   _____

Thorazine _____

Nurse practitioner _____

PARENTAL INFORMATION AND INFORMED CONSENT STATEMENT
FOR ADMINISTRATION OF SPECIAL MEDICATION

Doctors have known about the condition called *hyperactivity* for over 40 years. During this period it has been referred to by several different names. One of the most recent names was *minimal brain dysfunction or MBD for short.* At the present time the name that most doctors use is *attentional deficit disorder* or ADD for short.

Because children with this condition have great difficulty paying attention and sitting still, they have significant learning and behavior problems in school. In some cases, medication is required. When medication is recommended, it is because the doctor feels that the child can be expected to have serious problems with learning or behavior in school.

In the treatment of any condition *no effective medication is completely risk-free;* one must balance the risks of not prescribing against the risks of possible side effects of the medication. There are three medications commonly used today: Cylert, Dexedrine, and Ritalin. They all have similar actions, side effects, and risks. The possible side effects can be divided into three categories: frequent, occasional, and rare.

Frequent: Loss of appetite and delay in weight gain or actual weight loss. Since most children only take this medication during school days, they make up any weight loss on holidays and during the summer months.

This side effect is not considered serious and, unless it is marked, is not a reason for withholding medication.

Occasional:

1. Drowsiness
2. Upset stomach
3. Headache
4. Insomnia
5. Increased blood pressure
6. Aggravation of hyperactivity
7. Nervousness

These side effects can usually be eliminated by a reduction in dose or a change in the time the medicine is given. If persistent, the medicine may be stopped.

Rare

1. Addiction
2. "Zombie" or trance states

These two side effects occur only when excessive dosage is given, never when the medication is properly prescribed, administered, and monitored.

3. Tics or habit spasms

Children who already have involuntary twitching movements of the facial muscles, head, arms, or legs (tics) may become worse if these medications are used. Therefore, this type of medicine should *not* be used in children with tics.

For unknown reasons, tics tend to be familial; therefore, children who need medication but have close family members with tics should be watched very closely. At the first sign that tics may be developing, the medicine should be stopped. If children are not closely monitored, it has been estimated that tics may develop in about 1 out of 1,500 children taking this type medication.

I have read and understand the above statement and request that _____ receive medication for ADD.

Date _____   Signature _____
Father, mother, legal guardian
(Circle one)

DAILY LOG OF MEDICATION ADMINISTRATION

School _____   Month _____

Name	D.O.B.	Medication/dose	Time		Date					Date					Date					Date					Date				
			A.M.	P.M.	Mon.	Tues.	Wed.	Thurs.	Fri.	Mon.	Tues.	Wed.	Thurs.	Fri.	Mon.	Tues.	Wed.	Thurs.	Fri.	Mon.	Tues.	Wed.	Thurs.	Fri.	Mon.	Tues.	Wed.	Thurs.	Fri.

AB, absent; R, refused; NS, no show; DC, discontinued.

Guidelines for Completing

All students receiving medication at school, short term and/or long term, should be logged on this form.

Use a new form each month.

File completed forms in a file folder labeled Completed Record of Medication Administration and discard at the end of each school year.

Instructions:

A. *Medication column*
   1. *Write in name of medication on the top half of the medication/dose block.*
   2. *Dose is to be written in the lower half.*
   3. *Use one line for each medication to be given.*
   4. *When a student is receiving more than one medication, ditto marks may be used instead of rewriting the student's name.*

B. *Time column*
   1. *Write in exact time medication is to be given.*

   2. *To enter two different times in the A.M. and/or P.M. block, slash the square as follows:* 8/11   12/3

C. *Day of the week blocks*
   1. *Person administering the medication is to initial the appropriate block to indicate medication was given.*
   2. *Slash day block to initial different times medication was given.*
   3. *If medication is not given, enter the letter or letters that best describe the reason from the legend (right upper corner of form).*

D. *Columns not listed are self-explanatory.*

MEDICATION ENVELOPE

Name _____ D.O.B. _____

School _____ Grade _____ Year _____

Medication _____

Method of administration _____ Dosage _____

Time _____ Date Started _____

Doctor _____ Other info. _____

Date/Time/Signature   **Date/Time/Signature**

_____   _____

_____   _____

_____   _____

_____   _____

_____   _____

_____   _____

_____   _____

_____   _____

_____   _____

_____   _____

_____   _____

_____   _____

_____   _____

_____   _____

_____   _____

_____   _____

_____   _____

_____   _____

_____   _____

_____   _____

_____   _____

_____   _____

_____   _____

_____   _____

_____   _____

_____   _____

_____   _____

REQUEST FORM FOR _____ MEDICATION

Student's name _____ **D.O.B.** _____

School _____ **Grade** _____

Number of bottles, tablets, etc. _____

Date _____ **Nurse** _____

KWELL LOTION REQUEST FORM

Student's name _____ **D.O.B.** _____

School _____ **Grade** _____

Number of bottles (2 oz.) _____

Date _____ **Nurse** _____

FORMS FOR
NURSE'S REPORTS

In addition to the forms used to record daily activities, school nurses are often required to submit weekly, monthly, or annual reports that are compiled into district totals. Periodic campus reports are useful for several reasons:

1. Any campus reports that are unusually deviant from the norm of all campuses can be investigated.
2. A record is available to justify the health program. Some programs may, due to lack of budget, be discontinued if administrators are not aware of the benefits of the program.

Almost all school districts, even those with minimal health programs, use some type of the reporting forms found in this section. Some forms are specifically designed for professional school nurses; others will be more easily adapted for use by health aides.

Health program directors will find a variety of reporting forms to fit the needs of their district.

SCHOOL NURSE PRACTITIONER REPORTING WORKSHEET

The School Nurse Practitioner Reporting Worksheet is for use by school nurse practitioners or nurses trained in physical assessment who perform screening or individual physical exams. Some obvious abnormalities, of course, are referred directly to the family physician. Other subtle or questionable abnormalities can be checked out with the school consulting physician prior to referral, thus saving the family a visit to the doctor.

SCHEDULE OF NURSE'S WORK

The Schedule of Nurse's Work provides the nurse with the means for accurate scheduling of work to be done and gives a clear account of what has been done. For substitute nurses and in team staffing patterns, the schedule work plan is essential. All nurses are encouraged to provide the building principal with a copy of the completed form to facilitate integration of health service activities into the total school program.

NURSE'S DAILY SCHEDULE OF ACTIVITIES

The Nurse's Daily Schedule of Activities is a ten-day forecast of activities to be accomplished during the school day. It reflects planning with classroom teachers and students and allows the nurse and nurse assistants to work with a known student population.

NEED ASSESSMENT INSTRUMENT

In the development of new health programs, as well as in the evaluation of existing programs, the Need Assessment Instrument is useful to obtain input from health service as well as other educational personnel. Specific needs for new programs can then be seen and listed in order of importance.

TELEPHONE CONVERSATION RECORD

The Telephone Conversation Record helps the school nurse record useful information from telephone conversations. These forms can be included in the student records or reports.

RECORD OF CLINIC VISITS

The Record of Clinic Visits indicates the cause and frequency of an individual student's visit to the health clinic. It is used to record health room visits at each school building, as well as keep a record of children who make frequent visits.

MONTHLY TRAVEL REPORT

The Monthly Travel Report is submitted by the school nurse for reimbursement when traveling from campus to campus during the scheduled school day. The form should be completed by the nurse and signed by the local building principal prior to submitting it to the central office.

CLINIC STUDENT ROSTER

Prepared by _____   **School** _____

Date	Time		Rm., Teacher/ Advisor	Student	Service rendered
	In	Out			

HEALTH ROOM REPORT ON PUPIL CONTACTS

Date	Time In	Out	Name Last	First	Back to class	First aid	Temperature	Conference	Rested	Telephone call	Sent home	Parent came	Nurse took home	Referred doctor	Vision screened	Hearing test	Reason

NURSE'S ANNUAL STATISTICAL SUMMARY

19___ to 19___

School Grade									
Enrollment									
Health appraisals									
Growth									
Height and weight									
Dental									
Inspections									
Referrals									
Vision									
Pupils tested									
Pupils retested									
Pupils referred									
Received care									
Teacher notification									
Color perception									
Boys tested									
Boys failed									
Teacher notification									
Hearing									
Pupils tested									
Pupils retested									
Failed threshold									
New cases									
Known cases									
Referred for care									
Received care									
Teacher notification									
Scoliosis screening									
Pupils screened									
Pupils rescreened									
Pupils referred x-ray									
Pupils diagnosed									
Pupils to follow									
Immunization program									
Notices mailed									
Pupils excluded									
Immunizations given									
Special education programs									
Screening assessment									
Medical update									
Health/development history									
Neuro evaluation									
Physical assessment									
School guidance meetings									
IEP meetings									
Annual Reviews									
Health office (total—not grade level)									
Student visits									
Health assessment									
Health counseling									
Medical/dental referral									
Other referral									
Contagious disease control									
Pupils inspected									
Pupils excluded									
Medications at school									
Accidents reported									
Physical/sexual abuse reported									

NURSE'S ANNUAL STATISTICAL SUMMARY
Page 2

_____
Year

_____   _____
                    School   Nurse

Examples of outstanding health problems referred or monitored. (Numbers of each are not necessary.)

1. _____
2. _____
3. _____
4. _____
5. _____
6. _____
7. _____
8. _____
9. _____
10. _____
11. _____
12. _____
13. _____
14. _____
15. _____
16. _____
17. _____
18. _____
19. _____
20. _____
21. _____
22. _____

Health Education Projects

Instructions: Please indicate and describe kinds of health education projects you have initiated and/or supported during the year. Topics may have included bulletin boards, cleanliness and grooming, dental health, family life education, first aid, narcotics, alcohol and tobacco, nutrition, parent education, physical fitness, weight control, and/or others.

_____

_____

_____

_____

_____

_____

_____

Professional Conferences/Meetings Attended

_____

_____

_____

Suggestions for Improvement of Health Services

_____

_____

_____

_____

_____

_____

_____

_____
Nurse's signature

_____
Principal's signature

_____
School

_____
Date

SCHOOL NURSE PRACTITIONER REPORTING WORKSHEET

School _____   S.N.P. _____

Name	Date Room	Defects (N.P.'s findings)	Date	M.D. comments

SCHOOL NURSING PERIOD ACTIVITY REPORT AND SUMMARY SHEET

Dates covered _____   No. nurse aides _____
          (six-week reporting period)

School _____   Total visits to school _____

Enrollment _____   Average hours per visit _____

I. Health supervision	No. pupils	No. ref.	Referrals completed		
			Valid ref.	Rec'd Tx.	Over ref.
Physical assessment					
Health counseling					
Major illness					
Minor illness					
Emergency					
First aid					
Emotional					
Meds. supervision					
Special procedure					
Child abuse					
Comm. disease					
Other					
II. Screening					
Vision					
Hearing					
Weight and Height					
Scalp and skin					
Blood pressure					
Dental					
Scoliosis					
Reportable disease					
TB skin test					
Other					

III. Health activities	Students	Classes	Parents	Staff	Community
Health teaching					
Health conference					

IV. Staff development	No.	Hrs req.
Orientation, self/others		
Supervision		
Class prep. time		
Staff meetings		
Professional meetings		
Professional growth		
Inservice		
V. Others		
Home visits		
Community meetings		
School-sponsored meetings		
Field Trips—sponsored		

Other activities:

Signature and title

176

MONTHLY SUMMARY OF HEALTH SERVICES

Date _____

School _____

Nurse/clerk _____

Screening

	Number served	Number referred	Follow-up information			
			Received care	Over referred	Outcome unknown	No action
Vision						
Hearing						
Scoliosis						
Height and weight						
Pediculosis, scabies						
B/P Student						
Adult						
Physical exam.						
Dental						
Other						
Total						

Special Education

Preassessment _____   Staffings _____

Health assessments _____   Child abuse _____

Health Education

Number of classes _____   Number of students _____

Other groups—teacher, PTA, etc. _____   Materials/counsel provided _____

Student Contacts

	Number served	Number referred	Received care	No action
Illness				
Injuries				
Consultation				
Total				

Other Activities

Parent contacts _____   Contact with outside agency _____

Home visits _____   Conferences with school staff _____

Medications _____

MONTHLY SUMMARY TASK-TIME REPORT

Date_____School_____Prepared by_____

Time spent in these activities this month:

	No.	Hours	Unmet requests	
1. Education services			No.	Tot. Est. Time
a. Health education, preparation				
b. Health education, preparation For whom, what group? _____				
_____				
_____				
2. Health Services				
a. Program health services (screening, etc.)				
b. Encounters with students				
Health assessments _____				
Student consultation _____				
First aid _____				
Acute illness _____				
c. Teacher consultation				
d. Parent consultation				
e. Preceptor consultation				
f. Referral procedures				
g. Staffing conferences				
h. Record keeping				
i. Clinic activities not already recorded (including Teacher Consultations and Home Visits)				
3. Administrative and management				
a. Staff training (training of health clerks, etc.)				
b. Health clerk supervisor/consultation				
c. Travel				
d. Administrative				
e. Continuing education/inservice training				
4. Other (specify):				

Nurse: Time spent at school A (no. of hours) _____

         Time spent at school B (no. of hours) _____

         Time spent at school C (no. of hours) _____

         Time spent at school D (no. of hours) _____

         Total time (in hours) for month _____

MONTHLY ACTIVITY REPORT

Month	Sept.	Oct.	Nov.	Dec.	Jan.	Feb.	Mar.	Apr.	May	TOTAL
Clinic visits										
Emergency to another school										
Hospital emergency										
Home visits										
No. urine										
Grade Early childhood										
No. referred										
Grade other levels										
No. referred										
No. hematocrit										
Grade E.C.										
No. referred										
Grade other levels										
No. referred										
No. blood pressures										
Grade 6										
No. referred										
Grade 9										
No. referred										
Grade other levels										
No. referred										

Month	Sept.	Oct.	Nov.	Dec.	Jan.	Feb.	Mar.	Apr.	May	TOTAL
No. heights and weights										
Grade K										
No. referred										
Grade 1										
No. referred										
Grade 3										
No. referred										
Grade 6										
No. referred										
Grade 9										
No. referred										
Grade other levels										
No. referred										
No. immunized										
No. hearing tests										
No. vision tests										

School _____   R.N. _____

SCHEDULE OF NURSE'S WORK

Week	Monday	Tuesday	Wednesday	Thursday	Friday
First					
Second					
Third					
Fourth					
Fifth					
Sixth					

NURSE'S DAILY SCHEDULE OF ACTIVITIES

Date	Class	First period	Second period	Third period	Fourth period	Fifth period	Sixth period	Seventh period	Eighth period	Ninth period	Tenth period	Eleventh period	Twelfth period	

Notes

NEEDS ASSESSMENT INSTRUMENT

Instructions: To plan health service activities to best serve you, we need your help! This survey lists 30 possible health service areas. Please respond to each item. In the columns on the left, mark an X in the box that best describes how important the service is. In the column on the right, mark an X in the box that best describes to what degree you believe service is being covered. Please mark a response in the left column and the right column for each of the 30 areas.

Name of school _____ Date _____

Position of person filling out survey (e.g., principal, teacher, nurse) _____

Number of days/week there is school nurse coverage _____

Importance					Coverage provided				
No	Little	Moderate	Very	**Service area**	Don't know	Not covered	Little coverage	Moderate coverage	Fully covered
				Written policies and procedures for district for school health services.					
				Written job description for school nurse.					
				Guidelines for types of health observations to be referred to nurse by school personnel.					
				Health information obtained on all new students.					
				School notified by parents of students with major or chronic health problems.					
				School personnel notified by nurse of students with major or chronic health problems, follow-up to see that needs are met.					
				Health screening program **Vision**					
				Hearing					
				Scoliosis					
				Height and weight					
				Dental					
				Office personnel role in *minor* first aid and sending sick students home.					
				School nurse role in *minor* first aid and sending sick students home.					
				School nurse role in relation to emergency medical care.					

Importance					Coverage provided				
No	Little	Moderate	Very	Service area	Don't know	Not covered	Little coverage	Moderate coverage	Fully covered
				School nurse obtaining health assessments on all students staffed by Handicapped Children's Educational Act.					
				School nurse attending staffings for interpretation of student's health needs and the educational significance.					
				School nurse provides feedback to school personnel on referrals they made.					
				Home visits by school nurse on students when indicated by health concerns.					
				School nurse role in counseling with students for drug abuse, pregnancy, child abuse, unwed mothers, difficult home situations, etc.					
				School nurse role in counseling with students for their health concerns and/or major health problems.					
				Role of school nurse in assisting school personnel in developing health education curriculum.					
				Role of school nurse in teaching health education in classroom.					
				Need for having a school nurse in each building while school is in session.					
				Inservice held annually by nurse with the teachers on how to handle health problems and emergencies in the school setting.					
				School personnel prepared to recognize signs of suspected communicable or nuisance disease.					
				School Immunization Law initial paperwork the responsibility of the school secretary.					
				School nurse doing follow-up on immunizations required for immunization law.					
				Local doctor's and dentist's involvement in planning school health programs.					

Importance					Coverage provided				
No	Little	Moderate	Very	Service area	Don't know	Not covered	Little coverage	Moderate coverage	Fully covered
				Local public health personnel involvement in planning school health programs.					
				Importance of school nurse having a Type E teaching certificate as required by Teacher Certification Act of 1975.					
				Inservice training available to school nurse.					
				Public health officer makes the decision when there is an epidemic and the school should be closed.					
				School health office is available in every school.					
				Individual health records available on all students.					
				Privacy for health assessments and counseling.					
				One cot available for every 400 students.					
				Telephone available for confidential health conversations.					
				Health clerks for minor first aid, school immunization law, basic screening, routine paperwork.					

TELEPHONE CONVERSATION RECORD

Conversation with _____

Date _____

_____A.M.

☐ I called party   ☐ Party called me   Time _____P.M.

Subject discussed:

_____
Signature

RECORD OF CLINIC VISITS

Grade _____

_____

_____

Telephone no. _____

_____
Last name   First   Middle   Birthdate

Date	Time In	Out	Sent to school nurse because	Condition noted and action taken by nurse

MONTHLY TRAVEL REPORT
(IN LIEU OF SCHEDULED ALLOWANCE)

Employee _____ |_|_|_|-|_|_|-|_|_|_|_|
Name   Social security number

School/department _____ _____ _____
Name   Box no.   Month/year

Record of transportation and duties performed

Day of month	Locations visited, people contacted, and official duties performed*	Leave		Arrive		Miles traveled	Fares paid*†
		Hour Min.	Mileage meter	Hour Min.	Mileage meter		

*Each location visited must be recorded on a separate line.
†Receipts required.

187

MONTHLY TRAVEL REPORT
Page 2

Record of transportation and duties performed

| Day of month | Locations visited, people contacted, and official duties performed* | Leave | | Arrive | | Miles traveled | Fares paid*† |
		Hour Min.	Mileage meter	Hour Min.	Mileage meter		

Forward to controller with payment voucher at the end of each month.

(1) Car mileage _____ (miles) at ____¢ per mile $ _____

(2) Fares paid $ _____

Monthly travel expense (1 + 2) $ _____

Year-to-date total (includes this month) $ _____

I certify that the above expenses are true and correct and were incurred by me in the performance of my official duties in accordance with policies of my Board of Education.

Approved by _____   _____
                    Supervisor   **Employee**

188

ANNUAL SUMMARY OF CHRONIC ILLNESS

Annual report _____ _____ _____ _____ School year _____ – _____
School   Address   District   County

Information provided by _____ _____   SNP ☐   BSN ☐   RN ☐   LPN ☐   Other _____
Name   Title   Check appropriate box

Total school population served_____ _____
Total students   Total schools

Chronic Illness Monitoring

	Number of students known with condition (do not include those listed as newly diagnosed)	Number of students newly diagnosed this year	Number of days lost from school due to this illness	Comments
Anorexia/bulemia				
Cerebral palsy				
Asthma				
Cystic fibrosis				
Diabetes				
Emotional problems				
Epilepsy				
Heart disease				
Hemophilia/bleeding disorder				
Juvenile rheu. disease				
Malignant disease				
Muscular dystrophy				
Renal disease				
Substance abuse				
ADD treated with medication				
Other				

Adolescent Pregnancy

Number of pregnant girls less than 18 years of age	Number starting prenatal care	
Elementary _____	Trimester 1 _____	Number delivered _____
Jr. high _____	Trimester 2 _____	Number of low-birth-weight babies (below 5½ lb) _____
High school _____	Trimester 3 _____	Number of abortions _____
	Number of dropouts due to pregnancy _____	

189

ANNUAL SUMMARY OF CHRONIC ILLNESS
Page 2

Other Programs

Screening and Prevention Programs

	Number screened	Number referred	Nursing intervention/ nursing monitoring	Examined by physician/treated	No treatment needed	Number of referrals not complete	Lost to follow-up
Anemia							
Hypertension							
Scoliosis							
Tuberculosis							
Height and weight — Overweight > 95%ile							
Underweight < 5%ile							

Instructions: Report only those accidents resulting in medical care or loss of one-half or more days of school.

Type of Accident	Bus	Bike	Classroom	Freeplay	P.E. Class	Sports practice	Official game
Head injury (concussion, etc.)							
Back injury							
Eye injury							
Fracture							
Sprain or strain							
Superficial injury (abrasion, contusion, laceration)							
Other (specify)							

Number of students on daily medication _____

PRN Medication _____

Number of child/sexual abuse cases reported _____

Number of home visits _____

Number of employee health evaluations _____

Number of consultations

Parent _____

P.M.D. _____

Faculty _____

Number of nursing procedures on handicapped or chronically ill children

Other Please List

Caths _____ _____

Stoma _____ _____

R.O.M. _____ _____

Feeding _____ _____

190

FORMS FOR PARENT INFORMATION, NOTIFICATION, AND RELEASE OF INFORMATION

HEALTH SERVICES PROVIDED BY SCHOOL

The Health Services Provided by School informs parents of the benefits of the health services provided by the school nurse to gain their support and cooperation. A copy of this sheet is given to each child who registers as a new student in this particular school district.

SAMPLE LETTER ABOUT HEALTH SERVICE ACTIVITIES

The sample letter is for communicating an account of available health service activities and the nurse's schedule to parents. Nurses are encouraged to offer assistance to their principals in adapting this information to each school and publishing it in a PTA newsletter sent to each parent or by individual notice to parents at the beginning of the school year.

APPOINTMENT SLIP

The Appointment Slip is used to advise parents of a nurse-initiated conference at school regarding a student's health problem. Nurses should advise the principal of this request for a parent conference. They may also want to indicate to the parents that the conference is of a nonemergency nature.

HEALTH SERVICES PROVIDED BY SCHOOL

Dear Parents,

Good health and good learning go together! To help your child stay healthy, many health services are available at school at no cost.

1. Screening physical examinations
2. Blood test to check for anemia
3. Eye tests (vision screening)
4. Immunizations
5. Urine test to check for protein and sugar
6. Hearing tests
7. TB skin tests
8. Scoliosis screening

A. State law requires that all students attending school have the following immunizations:
   1. DTP (diphtheria-tetanus-whooping cough) *or*
   2. DT (diphtheria, tetanus)
   3. Polio
   4. Measles
   5. Rubella
   6. Mumps

   You must show the school nurse a *written* record of your child's immunizations, or your child may get the immunizations from your family doctor, health department clinic, or school nurse.

B. **Eye test**
   State law requires that all students enrolled in school for the first time, or who are new students in our district, have an eye test by a vision specialist or a school nurse. You may present a written record of your child's eye test, or the school nurse will do the test.

C. **Medicines**
   If your child needs to take medicine during school hours, please talk to the school nurse or principal to make the necessary arrangements. Students are not allowed to carry or have medicines on their person.

D. **Emergency care**
   Your permission is required to obtain medical help for your son or daughter should he or she become seriously injured or ill while at school. Please sign the back side of the student registration data form and give your school principal a telephone number where you or a relative can be reached.

E. **Dental Services**
   A dental van visits the school at selected intervals. A dentist and dental hygienist provide a wide range of dental services for children who have no other access to dental care. Parental permission is required.

_____   _____   _____
School   Nurse   Telephone

HEALTH SERVICE ACTIVITIES LETTER
(English)

Date _____

Dear Parent:

All students in the district have access to services provided by a staff of professional school nurses who work under the direction of a school physician. Services available to your student include

—**First Aid for Illness or Injury**
In the event of a serious accident or other emergency, every effort is made to contact the parent immediately. When parents cannot be contacted, an emergency ambulance is called and the student is taken to an appropriate medical facility accompanied by an adult from the school.

—**Control of Communicable Diseases**
Immunization protection is monitored at appropriate intervals, and when needed, skin and scalp screening is done. Special monitoring and management procedures are maintained for control of other contagious diseases.

—**Health Screening**
Including vision, hearing, height, weight, scoliosis, blood pressure, and in some cases, chest and heart assessment will be done at age-appropriate intervals to identify suspected health problems.

Parents will be notified of student immunization needs and other acute care or health maintenance needs that require assessment and follow-up by the family doctor or other health care provider.

Our school nurse, Ms. _____, is in our building every week on

_____.
(building day(s))

You and your child are encouraged to share concerns or problems relevant to your child's health with the school nurse. If you need information about a specific health problem, help with locating or gaining access to health care facilities or provider resources, or perhaps adjustment in your child's school environment because of health needs (including in-school medication and other special procedures), your building nurse should be contacted.

Sincerely,

Principal

HEALTH SERVICE ACTIVITIES LETTER
(Spanish)

Fecha _____

Estimados Padres:

Todos los alumnos del distrito tienen acceso a los servicios facilitados por enfermeras profesionales que trabajan bajo la dirección del médico de la escuela. Los servicios disponibles para su estudiante incluyen:

Primeros Auxilios para Enfermedad o Accidente
En caso de accidente u otra emergencia, se hará todo el esfuerzo posible para notificar a los padres inmediatamente. Cuando no se pueda localizar a los padres se llamará a la ambulancia y el alumno será llevado a un centro médico adecuado acompañado por un adulto de la escuela.

Control de Enfermedades Contagiosas
La protección acerca de inmunizaciones es controlada a intervalos apropiados y cuando sea necesario se harán exámenes de la piel y del cuero cabelludo. Observaciones y tratamientos especiales son mantenidos para control de otras enfermedades contagiosas.

Exámenes de Salud
Incluyendo vista, oídos, altura, peso, escoliosis, presión arterial y en algunos casos del pecho y del corazón, se harán a intervalos de acuerdo con la edad del estudiante, para identificar problemas sospechosos de salud.

Los padres serán notificados acerca de las inmunizaciones que el alumno necesite así como cualquier otro tratamiento o mantenimiento de salud que necesite de parte de su familia o del doctor.

Nuestra enfermera, _____, está en nuestro edificio cada semana el
_____.
(dia(s) en el edificio)

Animamos a usted y a su hijo/hija a compartir cualquier preocupación o problema concerniente a la salud de su hijo/hija con la enfermera de la escuela. Si necesita información sobre algún problema de salud, ayuda en localizar alguna clínica de salud, o ajustes en el ambiente escolar de su hijo/hija debido a sus necesidades especiales (incluyendo darle medicinas dentro de la escuela o algunos otros procedimientos), debe comunicarse con la enfermera local.

Sinceramente,

Director

STUDENT RECORDS RELEASE AUTHORIZATION

To _____

_____

I hereby authorize and request you to release to
(school address)

The complete medical records in your possession concerning the evaluation and/or treatment of _____
_____ **during the period from** _____ **to** _____.

Name of parent/guardian _____

Date of birth _____ **Telephone** _____

Address _____

_____

Signature _____ **Date** _____
(If relative, state relationship.)

Witness _____ **Date** _____

Initiated by _____

EMPLOYEE RECORDS RELEASE AUTHORIZATION

To _____

_____

I hereby authorize and request you to release to
                              (school address)

The complete medical records in your possession concerning my evaluation and/or treatment during the

period from _____ **to** _____.

Name of employee _____

Date of birth _____ **Telephone** _____

Address _____

_____

Signature _____ **Date** _____
                   (If relative, state relationship.)

Witness _____ **Date** _____

Initiated by _____

INTERAGENCY REFERRAL

Student

Student's name _____ Birthdate _____ Gr. _____ Rm. _____

Address _____ Phone _____

School attending _____

Parent Consent

Parent authorization: I hereby consent to an exchange of medical information between the school district

and _____
                                    (Physician/clinic/agency/hospital)

concerning my child, _____, in order to enhance the treatment
                                    (Child's name)

and follow-up of the condition for which he/she is referred.

Signature of parent _____ Date _____

Referral

Name and address of physician, hospital, clinic/agency:

Data base/instructions given:

_____ Date _____
School nurse/SNP

Instructions: Please complete the reply section and return white copy in self-addressed envelope to the school nurse. Thank you.

Physician Reply

Findings or recommendations:

Follow-up:

_____ Student to return to physician for recheck.

_____ Student referred to another physician, clinic, or agency for further care or assistance.

_____ Student referred to school nurse for monitoring of problem.

To assist us in evaluating our services, please check where appropriate:

_____ Condition properly referred.

_____ Condition did not necessitate referral. Reason: _____

_____

_____

Signature of physician _____ Date _____

RETURN TO:
School:
Address:

AUTHORIZATION FOR RELEASE OF INFORMATION
TO SCHOOL DISTRICT

I, _____, hereby authorize

(Parent or legal guardian)

_____ to release the following

Information pertaining to _____

(Name)

Birthdate _____

Specify information _____

_____

_____

_____

Send to _____

Signature _____   Witness

Date _____   Date

AUTHORIZATION FOR RELEASE OF INFORMATION
FROM SCHOOL DISTRICT

I, _____

(Parent, legal guardian, or self—if at least 18 years of age)

hereby authorize the school district to release the following information pertaining to _____

(Name)

Birthdate _____

Specify Information _____

_____

_____

_____

Send to _____

_____
Witness

Signature

_____
Date

Date

REFERRAL FORM
(Confidential)

Instructions: Use typewriter or ballpoint pen; press firmly.

From	To
Sender and phone number	Attention:

Patient or client			Sex
			☐ Male
Birthdate	Phone number	Case number	☐ Female

Address (Directions if needed)	Name of parent or spouse

Patient Information (See Instructions)

Date _____ Authorized signature _____
(Print or type name and title.)

Consent

Permission is hereby granted to release pertinent medical and social information on the above-named patient or client.

Date _____ Signature _____

Reply

Date _____ Signature _____

RECORDS RELEASE AUTHORIZATION

To _____

_____

_____

I hereby authorize and request you to release to

_____

(Current school district)

_____

_____

The complete medical records in your possession concerning my evaluation and/or treatment during the period from

_____ **to** _____.

Name of patient _____

Date of birth _____ **Telephone** _____

Address _____

_____

Signature _____ **Date** _____

(If relative, state relationship.)

Initiated by _____

GUIDELINES FOR LIVING WITH A HYPERACTIVE CHILD

1. **Accept the fact that your child is intrinsically overactive and energetic.** His hyperactivity is not intentional. Do not expect to eliminate the hyperactivity; just keep it under reasonable control. Don't try to change the energetic child into a quiet child or "model child." This will cause more harm than good. The hyperactive child needs a tolerant, patient, low-key parent.

2. **Provide outlets for the release of excess energy.** These children need daily outside activities such as running, sports, or long walks. A fenced yard helps. In bad weather he needs a recreation room or garage where he can do as he pleases without criticism. Hyperactivity may be allowed in these ways but it should not be needlessly encouraged. Adults should not roughhouse with these children. Siblings should be forbidden to say "Chase me, chase me" or to instigate other noisy play. Rewarding hyperactive behavior leads to its becoming the main style of interacting with people.

3. **Keep the home existence organized.** Household routines help the hyperactive child accept order. Mealtimes, chores, and bedtime should be kept as consistent as possible. Predictable responses by the parents to daily events help the child become more predictable.

4. **Avoid fatigue.** When hyperactive children are exhausted, their self-control often breaks down and their hyperactivity becomes worse.

5. **Avoid formal gatherings.** Settings where hyperactivity would be extremely inappropriate and embarrassing should be completely avoided. Examples of this would be church, restaurants, etc. After the child develops adequate self-control at home, these situations can gradually be introduced.

6 **Maintain firm discipline.** These children are unquestionably difficult to manage. Rules should be formulated mainly to prevent harm to themselves or others. Aggressive behavior and attention-getting behavior should be no more accepted in the hyperactive child than in the normal child. The family needs a few clear, consistent, important rules, with other rules added at the child's own pace. Parents must avoid being after the child all the time with negative comments like "Don't do this" and "Stop that."

7. **Enforce discipline with nonphysical punishment.** The family must have an "isolation room" or "time-out place" to back up their attempts to enforce rules, if a show of disapproval doesn't work. This room can be the child's bedroom. The child should be sent there to "shape up" and allowed out as soon as possible. Without an isolation room, overall success is unlikely. Physical punishment should be avoided in these children since we want to teach them to be less aggressive, rather than make aggression acceptable. These children need adult models of control and calmness.

8. **Stretch his attention span.** Increased attention span and persistence with tasks can be taught to these children at home. The child can be shown pictures in a book, and if he is attentive, he can be rewarded with praise and a hug. Next, the parent can read stories to him. Coloring pictures can be encouraged and rewarded. Games of increasing difficulty can gradually be taught to the child, starting with building blocks and progressing eventually to dominoes, card games, and dice games. Matching pictures is an excellent way to build a child's memory and concentration span. The child's toys should not be excessive in number, for this can worsen his distractibility.

9. **Protect the child against any overreaction by school or neighbors.** If he receives a reputation for being a "bad kid," it is important that this doesn't carry over into his home life. At home, the attitude that must prevail is that he is a *"good child* with excess energy." It is extremely important that his parents don't give up on him. He must *always feel accepted* by his family. As long as he has this, his self-esteem and self-confidence will survive.

10. **Periodically get away from it all.** Parents must get away from the hyperactive child often enough to be able to tolerate him. Exposure to some of these children for 24 hours a day would make anyone a wreck. When the father comes home, he should try to look after the child and give his wife a deserved break. A babysitter two afternoons a week and an occasional evening out with her husband can salvage an exhausted mother.

11. **Medication may be necessary.** No parent wants to give medication when they think it's not necessary—neither do physicians. However, there are some cases in which medication is helpful and a controlled trial is perfectly safe. It can be just as harmful to withhold needed medication as it is to give too much of it.

APPOINTMENT SLIP
(English)

_____ School _____ Date

Dear _____

It is important that I discuss with you a problem relating to the health of your child, _____

_____.

Please meet me at the school on _____, _____, _____ **A.M.**
P.M.

Or telephone me at _____ **between** _____ **A.M.**
P.M.

Check below if I may or may not expect you at this time and return this slip to me.

_____

Nurse

☐ **I will be at the school at the indicated time.**

☐ **I am unable to be at the school at the indicated time.**

Date _____ Signed _____

Parent

AVISO DE CITA
(Spanish)

_____ Escuela _____ Fecha

Estimados padres _____

Es importante discutir con ud.(s) un problema relacionado con la salud de su niño/niña, _____

_____ .

Favor de venir a la escuela para tener una entrevista conmigo el

_____ , _____ , _____ **A.M.**
P.M.

o teléfonearme al _____ **entre** _____ **A.M.**
P.M.

Favor de marcar abajo si puede o no puede tener la intrevista y devolver éste aviso.

_____
Enfermera

☐ **Yo estare en la escuela al tiempo indicado**

☐ **Yo no puedo estar en la escuela al tiempo indicado**

Fecha _____ **Firma** _____
Padre/Madre

SCHOOL HEALTH RECORD UPDATE

Dear Parent:

In checking through your child's health record, I have found that some information is missing or incomplete. Please assist me by completing this form and have your child return it to school as soon as possible. This is needed for an update in your child's school health records.

Thank you for your cooperation. This information will help us to provide the best services for your child.

Sincerely,

School nurse

Please detach and return

Name _____ Grade _____ Date _____

Has there been any change in child's health during the past year? No _____ Yes _____

Hospitalization No _____ Yes _____ Explain _____

_____

Seen by a physician? No _____ Yes _____ Explain _____

_____

Illness or injury? No _____ Yes _____ Explain _____

_____

Current medication? Type _____ Dosage _____

Does medication need to be taken during school hours? No _____ Yes _____

If yes, please request medication permission form.

Additional immunizations? No _____ Yes _____ Please list _____

Other comments:

Completed by _____/ _____/ _____
                        Name   Date   Relationship to student

Current findings by nurse _____

_____

_____

Recommendations _____

_____

_____

_____

_____

_____

_____

_____   _____
     Date   **School nurse**

FORMS FOR
PHYSICAL EXAMINATIONS
AND NURSE ASSESSMENTS

PARENT PERMISSION TO EXAMINE

The purpose of the Parent Permission to Examine is to obtain parental permission for school personnel to perform a more detailed physical exam that may be required for a specific purpose, such as special education, special olympics, a vocational program, and so on.

The form must be signed by the parent before the examination. This is best done during a parental conference dealing with the child's placement in a special program. If a parental conference is not held, the form should be taken or sent to the parent, or the parent should come to the school (not carried home by the student).

**PARENTAL NOTIFICATION OF SCREENING
PHYSICAL EXAMINATION**

The Parental Notification of Screening Physical Examination notifies parents that physical exams will be conducted at school and gives them an opportunity to refuse the exam or to bring appropriate information to the school nurse, since many children have physical abnormalities that are already known to the parents.

Some school districts notify parents that screening physical examinations are going to be performed and ask the parents to notify the principal if they want their child excluded. Some districts only perform exams on children for whom they have received signed parental permission.

Districts in which the children need the exam usually receive back about half the notes they send to parents; therefore, they usually use parental notification rather than signed permission.

Some parents prefer their child not have a physical exam at school, choosing to use their family physician. (In the author's district, about 12,000 physical exams are done by the school annually; usually about five or six parents districtwide come to the principal with a request for an examination by the family physician.)

The parental notification form is intended for the principal to duplicate and send to parents of children who are scheduled for a screening physical exam. Each district should decide which grade levels will be screened; therefore, input from a medical consultant is helpful.

REFERRAL TO PHYSICIAN OF DISCOVERED ABNORMALITIES

The purpose of the Referral to Physician of Discovered Abnormalities is to ensure that each child with previously unsuspected physical abnormalities be seen by a physician.

If possible, the form should be given directly to the parent rather than sent home with the child so that parental questions and concerns can then be dealt with directly. This also eliminates the frequent loss of the form when sent home with the child. Furthermore, a child would not understand the implications of the findings and would become worried if asked to carry the message home.

MEDICAL REFERRAL/FOLLOW-UP FORM

The Medical Referral/Follow-Up Form is used in referring a child for medical diagnosis and care. The nurse signs the form with her degree indicated. Nurse assistants/nurse aides, principals, and/or others should complete the medical referral for emergency care of students acutely ill or injured when the nurse is not in the building. The person completing the referral signs the form and specifies the job title.

Nurse assistants/nurse aide staff should be reminded that student referrals to physicians and health care community are initiated only by the school nurse except in the case of acute illness or injury as described above.

If evaluation by a physician is required before returning to school, this information should be included on the form.

A duplicate copy of the form should be used by the nurse to follow up on the referral. If the student does not bring the completed referral to the clinic, the nurse should take measures to ascertain the current status. If the condition is still present, the nurse should take appropriate steps, such as calling the parent, making a home visit, or sending an appointment slip.

ANNUAL/MONTHLY REPORT OF SCREENING PHYSICAL EXAMS

The purpose of the Annual/Monthly Report of Screening Physical Exams is to record the results of the screening physical exams for each campus and compile a list of abnormalities found by grade level.

Physical examinations for school enrollment at various grade levels are mandated by some states and encouraged by others. In states in which the examination is legislatively required, some school districts require the parent to obtain the examination at their own expense or go to an urban health center that may be inexpensive or free. Some school districts provide the physical exam at the school at no expense to the parent. The exam may be performed by contract physicians or school nurse practitioners or physician's assistants; the last two work under a physician's supervision.

The results of the exam are usually recorded on the student health card and become part of the permanent record.

Many school districts also offer screening physical exams at no expense to parents even though there is no legislative requirement. This usually occurs in larger, older, inner-city school districts with many single-parent children. There is usually no reimbursement to the school district, although some have been able to work out arrangements with the Department of Human Services for Title XIX reimbursement.

The following report documents the *numbers* and *kinds* of abnormalities found at a single campus, thus proving the value of the service. It is helpful to have these figures because some people feel that the physical exam should be done on an individual basis in the doctor's office, rural or urban health center, or other medical facility and not as a screening procedure at school. However, many of the children in older inner-city districts have no real access to physicians, so school health screening programs provide these children with the only continuity of care they get.

REPORT OF INDIVIDUAL PHYSICAL EXAMINATION

The Report of Individual Physical Examination insures communication among parents, agencies, and physicians who are part of the child's health care team.

Some larger school districts have well-established diagnostic/appraisal centers, where educational diagnosticians, psychological associates, and psychologists perform more sophisticated educational, psychometric, and psychological testing. In some districts, a medical/nursing component has been added to perform medical histories, physical examinations, and developmental neurological examinations by physicians or school nurse practitioners.

This form can also be used by private physicians for feedback to the school regarding their examination of the student.

MEDICAL REPORT FROM SCHOOL

The information from the physical examination may be recorded on the Medical Report from School and shared with parents when appropriate. Nurse practitioners are encouraged to complete the form for an EPSDT screening report to parents.

MEDICAL REPORT

The Medical Report is given to parents of all students new to the district—K-1 plus upper grade new pupils. Physical and dental exams may not be required for new pupil enrollment, but should be encouraged.

The report gives detailed information regarding immunization enrollment requirements and may be offered to persons requesting such information. This form may also be used to transcribe pupil immunization information for students requesting a copy of immunization status. Immunizations are acceptable on any official medical record with proper physician/public health clinic verification.

PHYSICAL EXAMINATION FORM

The Physical Examination Form can be used for individual physical exams performed on the same student at various intervals. The form is usually used for a child with chronic health problems.

CONDITIONS REFERRED TO PHYSICIAN—ANNUAL REPORT

The Conditions Referred to Physician—Annual Report is used by each campus to list all the children referred to a doctor during the entire year, plus the number actually seen by a doctor. It gives a nurse a good idea of how effective the referral process is at any one campus.

MEDICAL/NEUROLOGICAL EVALUATION PACKET

The Medical/Neurological Evaluation Packet is a specialized form to be used by school nurse practitioners, physician's assistants, or appropriately trained professional school nurses working with a school physician. Its purpose is to have a detailed medical evaluation of children with severe learning and behavior problems that have an adverse effect on the child's academic achievement and/or social adjustment.

Proper completion of the form requires the school nurse to:

1. Consult with the student's teachers and counselor.
2. Record a complete medical history with emphasis on developmental, social, and cultural factors.
3. Perform a standard physical examination.
4. Do a developmental neurological examination.
5. Have sufficient knowledge of educational and psychometric testing to summarize the testing.

Some medical history forms consist of a detailed checklist on which parents, school nurses, or nurse practitioners can check off the appropriate box. Check-off lists are easier to use if personnel cannot be adequately trained in history-taking technique.

The developmental neurological exam sequence is not part of the form but is included to show how the reporting check sheet is derived.

The summary of psychometric tests should list the tests in use in any given school district. This form is to record tests done by educational diagnosticians or other educational personnel, but not by school nurses. The nurse then uses this form to summarize the testing data and submit it to the physician consultant.

PARENT PERMISSION TO EXAMINE

I, _____, hereby authorize _____
        Parent's name

_____ of the _____ School District,
        Title

Health Services Department, to perform a medical evaluation without cost on my child or ward,

_____, a student at _____ school.
        Child's name

Purpose of medical evaluation:

☐ Special education (evaluated by advanced nurse practitioner/physician assistant)[1]

☐ Health care maintenance (evaluated by registered nurse)[2]

☐ Other _____

Medicaid ☐ Yes   ☐ No   If yes, please give child's number _____

I understand that all reasonable precaution and care will be taken in giving the medical evaluation to my child. (See below for explanation of medical evaluation.) I have read and understand the explanation of the medical evaluation.

_____

Signature of parent/guardian

_____

Date

Home   **Work**

_____

Telephone number parent/guardian

[1] The examinations done by physician's assistance or nurse practitioners are directed and supervised by a licensed physician.

[2] Health maintenance examinations by registered nurses are supervised by nurse practitioners.

The medical evaluation consists of the history and physical examination.

The medical history should include information about major past health problems (physical and emotional) and their treatment, an orderly review of body systems, information about current and past special problems of other members of the family, and information about the child's academic achievements and school adjustment. The medical history in some cases will review practices that influence health either favorably or adversely (such as smoking, exercise, diet and sleep).

The physical examination consists of a measurement of the height, weight, and blood pressure; a complete examination of the head and neck; chest including the heart; lungs and breasts; abdomen; genitalia (if indicated); musculoskeletal system; and the nervous system.

PARENTAL NOTIFICATION OF SCREEN PHYSICAL EXAMINATION

Dear Parent:

The _____ School District, Department of School Health Services, offers, free of charge, a routine screening physical examination to students *once* when enrolled in prekindergarten, kindergarten, or first grade; again in the third grade; and/or upon special referral.

_____ Elementary School is scheduled to have its students receive a physical

examination the week of _____. If for any reason you do not want your child to receive this service, please notify the school principal.

_____   _____

Date   Principal

REFERRAL TO PHYSICIAN OF DISCOVERED ABNORMALITIES

To the parent or guardian of _____ D.O.B. _____
Student's name

As a result of the school Health Department's screening program the following conditions have been found:

_____
Date

_____
Date

_____
Date

_____
Date

☐ The conditions listed are *not* serious and it is *not* necessary to see your doctor immediately. At your next regular visit, ask about it. We suggest you have it checked no later than 3   6   9 months from now.   (Circle one)

☐ The conditions listed should be examined by your doctor as soon as possible.

If you need more information or need help in locating a doctor, feel free to call your school nurse.

_____
School nurse   Date

_____
School   Phone number

Doctors' Report to School Nurse (Please return as soon as possible.)

Findings and recommendations given to parents _____

_____

_____

Are any modifications of the school program indicated? If so, what? _____

_____

_____

Do you wish to see the child again? If so, when? _____

_____   _____
Physician's printed name   Physician's signature

_____   _____
Office telephone number   Date

A MULTIREFERRAL FORM

To the parent or guardian of _____

Last name   First name

_____

School   Grade

_____ law requires the schools to screen all students in grades _____ annually for vision and hearing. The law also requires that parents or guardians of students who fail the screening tests be notified of this fact. Other screening programs are conducted each year as a service to students.

The student mentioned above has failed the screening test indicated below. We recommend that you contact your family health care professional regarding his or her condition.

_____ Audiometric tests show probable loss of hearing.

_____ Eye tests indicate probable vision difficulty.

_____ Teeth inspection indicates probable need for dental care.

_____ Scoliosis screening test indicate possible spinal curvature.

_____ Other _____

Please come and talk to me at _____**School,**

at _____ **o'clock, on** _____ **regarding your child.**

Signed _____

School nurse

Please return this note telling us what has been done relative to this notice. Thank you.

_____

_____

_____

_____

_____

_____

_____

_____

_____

_____

_____

Date _____ **Signed** _____

Parent

SCHOOL HEALTH PROGRAM LETTER TO PARENT

School _____ Date _____

Name of child _____ Grade _____

Name of teacher _____

Dear Parent:

The teacher and I have noted the following condition(s) that we feel should be brought to your attention:

_____

_____

_____

_____

_____ _____ _____
       Principal   **Nurse**   **Phone**

The school would appreciate comments from you or your doctor regarding these signs if you feel the information would be helpful for the nurse or teacher.

Date _____

Parent's comments *or* doctor's diagnosis, treatment, and recommendations:

_____

_____

_____

_____

_____

_____

_____

_____

_____

_____

_____

_____ *or* _____
     Parent's signature   **Doctor's signature**

MEDICAL REFERRAL/FOLLOW-UP FORM

Dear Parent:

It is recommended that you take your child along with this form to your doctor/dentist for recommendations regarding the possible health problem indicated below. We are anxious to give you any assistance we can in getting your child's problem corrected. Your child's adjustment in school is likely to be improved by your early attention to this matter.

Your school nurse

Estimados Padres:

Es recomendado que usted lleve a su hijo/hija a ver a un médico/dentista para recibir recomendaciones acerca de los posibles problemas de salud indicados mas adelante. Haga favor de llevar este formulario con usted al visitar al médico/dentista. Estamos anciosos de darles cualquier asistencia que podamos en la correción del problema de su hijo/hija. El ajustamiento de su hijo/hija en la escuela probablemente mejorara a causa del la atención rapida de usted a este problema.

La enfermera de la escuela

Dear Doctor:

We have checked _____ (Name)

_____ (Home address) _____ (Home telephone) _____ (School) _____ (Grade)
who presents the following type of health problem:

Dental — Major trauma — Minor trauma — Illness/abnormality — Symptoms without signs — Vision — Hearing —
Other _____

Please indicate the 70 and prognosis of the condition you find and advise us of the need for any limitation of activity, prosthesis, special class, or any action we might well pursue to improve the health of this child.

Our observations are as follows: _____

_____

_____

_____

_____

_____

Date _____

Professional Opinion with Recommendations

_____

_____

_____

_____

_____

_____

_____

Full activity including P.E. No ☐   Yes ☐   If no, please check appropriate box below.

☐ Vigorous activities   ☐ Moderate activities   ☐ Mild activities

☐ Complete rest or exemption.   Date of return to full physical activity _____

Signature of doctor _____ Telephone _____ Date _____

Is there any specific time you wish to see this pupil again? Yes _____ No _____ When? _____

Please return to the school nurse or, if information is confidential, return in mail to director of School Health Services.

216

SCHOOL NURSE PRACTITIONER REFERRAL TO PHYSICIAN

This child has been seen by the school nurse and further assessed by the school nurse practitioner. The condition described below is of sufficient importance to warrant referral to the child's primary physician. Please complete the bottom half of this form and return to the address above. Feel free to call for further explanation or information.

Student's name _____ Date _____

School _____ D.O.B. _____

Referral to _____

Reason for referral _____

_____

_____

_____

Specific information requested from physician: _____

_____

_____

_____
School nurse practitioner

Response _____

_____

_____

_____

Suggestions for educational and/or physical classroom management, if any:

_____

_____

_____

_____

_____

_____

_____

_____

_____

_____

_____

_____   _____
Printed name   Signature

_____   _____
Office telephone number   Date

ANNUAL/MONTHLY REPORT OF SCREENING PHYSICAL EXAMS

School _____ Campus nurse _____

Date _____ _____ _____

Name of examiner   Title

Instructions: Fill in number of students with abnormalities.

	Pre-K	Kinder-garten	First grade	Third grade	Special Ed.	Other grade levels
No. examined						
No. with abnormality						
Tonsils						
Teeth						
Nonrefractive error Eye						
Ear						
Heart						
Posture						
Overweight						
Underweight						
Hernia						
Varicocele						
Hydrocele						
Undescended testicle						
Skin condition						
Gait disturbance						
Spine						
Miscellaneous (specify)						
Total abnormalities						

ANNUAL SCHOOL HEALTH SERVICES REPORT

Supervisory union _____

Year _____

School _____

Population _____

Grade level (check one)
Elementary ( )
Middle/Junior ( )
High ( )

	Total students	Receiving treatment	Referrals M.D.	Community agency	Other
Screening					
Vision					
Speech					
Hearing					
Blood pressure					
Throat culture					
Height and weight, obesity, undernutrition					
Posture					
Dental					
Interventions					
Accidents					
Complaints					
Alcohol counseling					
Substance abuse					
Mental health					
Nutrition					
Pregnancy					
Other*					
Conferences					
Parents					
School personnel					
Interagency					
Home visits					
Other*					

*Describe.

REPORT OF INDIVIDUAL PHYSICAL EXAMINATION

The student named below received a physical examination at the _____
today. Please transfer the information provided to the student's health card and complete any requested follow-up. You may use this form to respond to _____ concerning follow-up. If no follow-up is requested, please dispose of this form after information has been recorded on student's health record.

Student's name _____ D.O.B. _____ School _____

Date _____

Reason for exam _____

Nose _____	Blood pressure _____
Teeth _____	Head circumference _____
Tonsils _____	
Ears _____	Height _____
Heart _____	Weight _____
Lungs _____	Vision _____
Chest _____	Hearing _____
Spine _____	Other _____
Hernia _____	
Genitalia _____	

Comments:

Follow-up requested from campus nurse:

220

MEDICAL REPORT FROM SCHOOL

(In English)

Dear Parents:

_____ was examined at school today. The findings are as follows:

Weight _____ Height _____ Blood pressure _____ Urine _____

Vision: R _____ L _____ Hearing: R _____ L _____

Color vision _____

T.B. Skin test (R forearm) _____ To be read _____ Results _____

Physical exam Legend: V = normal; X = abnormal; ND = not done.

Skin/scalp _____ Abdomen _____

Eyes, ears, nose, throat_____ Genitalia _____

Mouth/teeth_____ Bones/joints/extremities _____

Chest _____ Neurological _____

Heart/circulation _____ Development _____

Comments_____

Referral _____

Signed _____ Title _____

Date _____ Telephone _____

(In Spanish)

Estimados Padres:
Hoy en la escuela se le hizo un examen a _____

Los resultados son los siguentes:

Peso _____ Estatura _____ Presion de sangre _____ Analisis de orina _____

Examen para la vista: R ____ L ____ Examen para oir: R ____ L ____

Segura a los colores: Normal/anormal _____

Prueba para el tuberculosis (brazo derecho): Fecha para interpretar _____ Resultados _____

Examen fisico marca: V = Normal; X = Anormal; NE = No se examina

Piel/cuero cabelludo _____ Abdomen _____

Ojos/oldos/Nariz/Garganta _____ Genitales _____

Boca/dientes_____ Huesos/coyunturas/brazos/piernas _____

Pecho _____ Neurologico_____

Corazon/circulacion _____ Desarrollo _____

Comentarios_____

Anormalidad que requiere atencion medica _____

Firmada_____ Titulo _____

Fecha_____ Telefono _____

MEDICAL REPORT

Dear Parent:
Student immunization and vision screening, as described below, are required by state law. The required information must be submitted to the school for student enrollment.

Pupil's name _____ Sex _____ Birthdate _____

School attended _____ Grade _____

I. Immunization requirements. *Must be validated* by physician's signature or health clinic stamp:

Diphtheria-tetanus Three doses vaccine with one since fourth birthday and every 10 years thereafter   Date ____   Date ____   Date ____

Poliomyelitis (to age 18 years) Three doses vaccine with one since fourth birthday   Date ____   Date ____   Date ____

Measles One dose vaccine since first birthday (since January 1968) or physician verified history of disease.   Date ____   or history of measles disease   Date ____

Rubella (to age 12) One dose vaccine   Date ____

Mumps One dose vaccine or physician verified history of disease on all students with birthdate on or after August, 1971.   Date ____   or history of mumps illness   Date ____

_____   _____   _____   _____
Name of physician (please print)   Date   Signature of physician   Phone

II. Vision screening requirement for all *students* not previously enrolled in a school within the state.
The required vision screening will be done by the district's School Health Services staff unless you submit test results over the signature of your examining doctor or make signed application for provisional enrollment with a pending appointment for examination (not to exceed 90-day grace period).

Vision examination by doctor
☐ A. Test results (current within 1 year) attached or submitted below
☐ B. Test results pending, appointment on___ Month _____ Day _____ Year _____
Date of appointment (within 90 days)

_____   _____
Parent signature   Date

Vision test results: Without glasses: R-20/____   _____
L-20/____   Signature of state-certified medical examiner

III. Physical examination (recommendations)

Skin/scalp _____ Abdomen _____

E.E.N.T. _____ Limbs _____

Mouth _____ Teeth _____ Bones and joints _____

Chest _____ Reflexes _____

Heart and circulation _____ Others _____

_____

_____

Does the school program need to be accommodated for this student? Explain:

_____

Comments/Impression _____

Date _____ Signed _____ M.D.   Telephone _____
D.O.

_____

IV. Dental report (recommended)

Pupil's name _____
Last   First   Middle
Please indicate type of dental care given.

Prophylaxis _____ Cavities filled _____ Operative _____ Orthodontics _____

What additional care do you plan for this child? _____

_____

Date _____ Signed _____ D.D.S.   Telephone _____

222

PHYSICAL EXAMINATION FORM

Instructions: Indicate abnormality by placing an "X" in the appropriate box.

Name _____

Date	Age	Temperature	Height	Weight	Head circumference	Blood pressure	General appearance	Nutritional status	Skin	Glands	Eyes	Ears	Mouth/throat	Nasopharynx	Teeth	Heart	Chest/lungs	Abdomen	Genitalia	Skeletal	Feet	Neurological	Date of Next Medical Examination	Signature

CONDITIONS REFERRED TO PHYSICIAN—ANNUAL REPORT

Campus _____ School year _____

	Number referred	Number seen by doctor		Number referred	Number seen by doctor
Orthopedic			**Eyes**		
Scoliosis			Refractive error Exophoria		
Gait disturbance			Esophoria		
Club foot			Ptosis		
Other			Other		
Genitourinary			**Miscellaneous**		
Cryptorchid			Umbilical hernia		
Hydrocele			Lungs (wheezing, URI)		
Phimosis					
Hypospadius			Tonsils		
Inguinal hernia			Deviated nasal septum		
Other			Enlarged lymph nodes		
Ear					
Otitis media			Pectus excavatum		
Foreign object in ear			Pectus carinatum		
Other			Torticollis		
Endocrine			Baker's cyst		
Goiter			Dermatitis		
Obesity			Other		
Other					
Cardiac					
Murmur					
Arrythmia					
Other					

FOLLOW-UP ON PHYSICIAN REFERRALS

Campus nurse _____   School _____

Name	Grade	Rm	D.O.B.	Date of assessment	Medical problem referred	Physician's diagnosis and recommendation	Date	Disposition of case
1.								
2.								
3.								
4.								
5.								
6.								
7.								
8.								
9.								
10.								
11.								
12.								
13.								
14.								
15.								
16.								
17.								
18.								
19.								
20.								
21.								
22.								
23.								
24.								
25.								
26.								
27.								
28.								
29.								

MEDICAL/NEUROLOGICAL EVALUATION (Short Form)

Name _____ Date _____

School _____ Class placement _____ D.O.B. _____

Reason for referral:

Significant historical factors (prenatal, natal, infancy, early childhood, family, social, school):

Language development:

Significant findings on physical exam: Audiometric _____ Vision (L) _____
(R) _____

Height _____% **Weight** _____% **Head circumference** _____% **Blood pressure** _____

Significant findings on developmental neurological exam:

MEDICAL/NEUROLOGICAL EVALUATION (Long Form)

Name _____ Date _____

School _____ Class placement _____ D.O.B. _____

Reason for referral (School social behavior, academic achievement, and brief statement of school's expectations from medical evaluation):

Interview history: (Prenatal, natal, neonatal, developmental milestones, early childhood development, past history, family history, social history, school history):

Informant

Instructions: To continue, use reverse side or additional paper.

MEDICAL/NEUROLOGICAL EVALUATION (Long Form)
Page 2

Physical Examination*

Weight ____	Height ____	Head circum. ____	B/P ____
General physique ____	Head ____	Facies ____	Teeth ____
Eyes ____	Ears ____	Nose ____	Throat ____
Heart ____	Lungs ____	Chest ____	Abdomen ____
Skin ____	Genitalia ____	Spine ____	Extremities ____

*O, normal; X, abnormal; NE, not examined.

Developmental Neurological Evaluation*

	Results (N-M-S)		Results (N-M-S)
1. Speech	_____	7. Block design	_____
2. Coordination	a b c d	8. Six-sticks	_____
3. Sequential finger-thumb	_____	9. Eye convergence	_____
4. Muscle tone	_____	10. Balance	a b c
5. Graphesthesia	_____	11. Choreiform movements	_____
6. Astereognosis	_____	12. Gait	_____

*N, normal; M, mild impairment; S, severe impairment results.

Summary and Suggestions

Evaluator _____ SNP, PA, RN   Approved by _____ M.D.

SOFT SIGN SCREENING

Name _____ Age _____ Grade _____

School _____

Hop on one foot, then the other: _____ Right _____ Left

Skip _____ (Note clumsiness and sequence.)

Feet together, hands outstretched _____ (Eyes open.)

Balance on one foot, then the other: _____ Right _____ Left

Heel to toe _____

Preferred hand _____ Preferred foot _____

Stand: Turn left _____ Turn right _____

Hand on ear: _____ Right _____ Left Hand on knee: _____ Right _____ Left

Eye tracking: _____ Preferred eye _____ Right _____ Left

Convergence _____

Identify given objects _____ (pen, paper clip, coins, eraser, key, etc.)

Write numbers 1–10:

Reproduce: ✛ ◯ △ ◇ ◇ ◈

Comments _____

_____

_____

_____

_____

_____

_____

_____

_____

_____

_____

DEVELOPMENTAL TESTING

Name _____ D.O.B. _____ School _____

Date of test

_____
1. **WISC, WAIS, WPPSI, WISC-R**
   Verbal

   Scaled Scores Performance

   a. Information _____   a. Picture completion _____

   b. Comprehension _____   b. Picture arrangement _____

   c. Arithmetic _____   c. Block design _____

   d. Similarities _____   d. Object assembly _____

   e. Vocabulary _____   e. Coding _____

   f. Digit span _____   f. Mazes _____

_____ 2. **Stanford-Binet**   M.A. _____

_____ 3. **Slosson Int. Test**   M.A. _____

_____ 4. **Columbia M.M.T.**   M.A. _____

_____ 5. **Peabody Picture Vocabulary**   M.A. _____

_____ 6. **DAP: DMA** _____   P.M.A. _____

_____ 7. **Bender DMA** _____   P.M.A. _____

_____ 8. **WRAT (grade level)**

   Reading _____ Spelling _____ Arithmetic _____

_____ 9. **PIAT (grade level)**

   Reading _____ Spelling _____ Arithmetic _____ Gen. _____

_____ 10. **Oral (instructional) reading level: Grade** _____

   Circle test used: Spacre   Durrell   Gray

   Other _____

_____ 11. **Handwriting sample or signature of student**

MA, mental age; DMA, developmental age; PMA, psychomotor age.

DEVELOPMENTAL NEUROLOGICAL EXAM

1. **Speech**
   a. Engage in sufficient informal conversation to assess clarity and intelligibility.
   b. Assess ability in child's best language.
   c. Only marked impairment (English or Spanish) counted as a soft sign.

2. **Coordination**
   a. Finger to nose—extend each arm laterally and touch 5 times with eyes open. Repeat with eyes closed.
      S—failure to touch tip nose at least three times with both hands, eyes closed.
   b. Pronation-supination-arm at side, elbow 90 degrees. Rotate palm 5 times. Both hands.
      S—movement both elbows 4 or more inches away from body.
   c. Foot taps—Seated in chair tap toe 10 times each foot with heel on floor.
      S—failure to sustain 6 consecutive toe taps with both feet.
   d. Heel shin—Seated, legs extended, heel-shin 2 times each foot.
      S—two or more losses or contact on four trials.

3. **Sequential finger-thumb**—Moderate speed. Sequence is index to pinky, pinky to index. Imitate examiner after each finger movement, both hands.
   S—two errors each hand (if not quickly corrected).

4. **Muscle tone**
   a. Arm
      1. Flap hand with forearm still and flexed 90 degrees.
      2. Plantar and dorsiflex wrist.
      3. Flex and extend elbow.
      4. Dorsiflex wrist and bend fingers back.
   b. Leg
      1. Hold thigh 90 degrees—swing lower leg.
      2. Test range of motion ankle.
         S—marked hypotonia or hypertonia in all four extremities.

5. **Graphesthesia**—Seated palms up, face averted.
   a. Identify written symbols: 2, 3, 8, A, C, R.
   b. Trace on palm of left hand 8, C, R.
   c. Trace on palm of right hand 3, A, 2.
      S—two failures each hand.

6. **Astereognosis**
   a. Show objects and ask to name: comb-key-quarter-penny.
   b. Seated, face averted. Identify each one with each hand.
      S—total of three tactile failures with accurate identification.

7. **Block design test**
   S—four failures in two hands.

8. **Six stick test**
   S—dropping four extra sticks, two hands.

9. **Eye convergence**
   S—complete failure of convergence, either eye.

10. **Balance**
    a. Standing—eyes closed, feet together, arms and fingers spread apart—30 sec.
       S—three or more back and forth body movements exceeding 1 inch in each direction.
    b. Hopping—ten times consecutively on each foot.
       S—failure to hop 5 times consecutively each foot.
    c. Tandem walk—10 steps heel to toe, arms at sides.
       S—failure to approximate heel-toe for at least 5 consecutive steps.

11. **Choreiform movements**—standing, feet together, arms outstretched, eyes closed. Observe small jerks or twitches in fingers, wrists, arms, shoulders
    S—ten twitches during 30 seconds.

12. **Gait**—walk back and forth (to and fro) 20 feet.
    S—any of four.
    a. A base wider than 10 inches.
    b. Failure to alternate flexion extension of knees smoothly.
    c. Absence of a heel-toe gait.
    d. Immobility of arms.

Adapted from Lawrence Taft, M.D., 1970.
N, normal; M, mild impairment; S, severe impairment.
3 or 4 soft signs at age 8 years constitutes a neurological abnormality. Only an "S" counts as a soft sign.

FORMS FOR PREGNANT STUDENTS

Pregnant teenagers have various options for their schooling during the last months of their pregnancy. They may choose to attend their regular school, drop out of school, or attend a special school (if the district provides one). Whatever the decision may be, medical care is required.

The following forms are useful for maintaining the various types of health records necessary for monitoring the progress of the pregnancy.

PREGNANT STUDENT HEALTH FORM

/		/	Yes/No	A N M-A I O
Student's last name	First	Middle	Married	Race (Circle one.)

Birthdate _____ **Age:** _____ | **Grade:** _____ **I.D.:** _____

Home telephone: _____ | **Business telephone: Mother** _____

| **Father** _____

Home address: _____ | **Notify in case of emergency:**

Name _____

Relationship _____

Phone _____

Home school _____ | **Credits/units** _____

Courses required

First quarter	Second quarter	Third quarter

Current grades

(Quarter)

	1	2	3
P.E.			

(Phone)

Approved _____
Principal's signature

_____
Advisory-guidance counselor's signature

_____
Student's signature

_____
Pupil personnel counselor's signature

I hereby grant permission to send my son/daughter to hospital via ambulance should it become necessary.

Signed _____
Parent/guardian

STATEMENT OF PHYSICIAN

_____
Student I.D. number

Name of student _____ / _____ / _____
　　　　　　　　　　　　　　Last　　　　　　　　First　　　　　　　Middle

Birthdate _____ / _____ / _____   _____
　　　　　Month　　Day　　Year　　　　　　　　　　　Home school site

Approximate date of delivery: _____

General medical evaluation is essentially normal except for pregnancy.

☐ Yes　　　　　　☐ No

If "No," please indicate health problems requiring additional precautions (diabetes, epilepsy, cardiac disease, asthma, etc.).

_____　　　_____
Name of physician (please print)　　　　　　　Signature of physician

Office phone _____ Office address _____

Date _____

235

HEALTH CARE MONITORING AND TEACHING RECORD
FOR PREGNANT STUDENT COUNSELING

Name _____ Date _____ Home school _____

Address _____ Home phone _____

Mother's name _____ Work phone _____

Father's name _____ Work phone _____

Age _____ D.O.B. _____ LMP _____ EDC _____ Week or month of pregnancy _____

Clinic or physician _____ Phone _____ First appointment _____

Routine prenatal health care visits are scheduled:
Every four (4) weeks up to 32 weeks (end of this period _____)
                                                    (Write in pencil.)

Every two (2) weeks up to 36 weeks (end of this period _____)
                                                    (Write in pencil.)

Then every week until delivery. Record dates for future medical prenatal care. When the appointment has been kept or changed, record the new date. Student to be seen by school nurse approximately midway between physician/clinic visits.

Medical prenatal appointments	School nurse prenatal appointments
1. ___ 2. ___ 3. ___ 4. ___ 5. ___	1. ___ 2. ___ 3. ___ 4. ___ 5. ___
6. ___ 7. ___ 8. ___ 9. ___ 10. ___	6. ___ 7. ___ 8. ___ 9. ___ 10. ___
11. ___ 12. ___ 13. ___ 14. ___ 15. ___	11. ___ 12. ___ 13. ___ 14. ___ 15. ___

Ongoing health problems:

Illness or injury:

Medications:

Hospitalizations:

Allergies:

School performance and attendance:

Review of systems:

  Skin

  Head

  Teeth

  Eyes

  ENT

  Pulmonary

  Cardiovascular (include present cardiac status)

  Gastroentestinal

  Genitourinary

  Musculoskeletal

  Neurological

  Psychological

  Endocrine (include present status)

  Hematopoietic (include bleeding abnormalities)

Family History:

Social History:

Past OB History (if applicable)

Gravida _____ Para _____ AB _____
No. of Pregnancies   No. of Live Babies

_____ Delivery: Vaginal _____ C-Section _____
Date

If C-Section, state reason: _____

Complications of pregnancy or delivery:

BP _____ Bleeding _____ Infection _____

Other:

BW _____ Health of baby _____

Present OB History

BP _____ Bleeding _____ Infection _____

Smoke _____ Drink alcohol _____ Use drugs _____

Other _____

HEALTH CARE MONITORING AND TEACHING RECORD
FOR PREGNANT STUDENT COUNSELING
Page 2

Prepregnant weight _____ **Date** _____ **Prepregnant BP** _____ **Date** _____

Monitoring—Counseling

Instructions: Inquire specifically about nutrition, headache, altered vision, abdominal pain, nausea, vomiting, bleeding, fluid or secretions from vagina, dysuria. Comment about health, nutrition, any classes re: labor, delivery, etc., being taken by student.

Date	Weight	Blood pressure	Visits with school nurse—comments	Learning module

Delivery _____ **Health of student** _____ **Baby's health and birth weight** _____
　　　　　　Date

Complications _____

Return to school _____ (usually two weeks after normal delivery, three weeks after C-section)
　　　　　　　　Date

Postpartum care _____

FORMS FOR
SCOLIOSIS

SCREENING FORMS

The forms in this section record all the results of a school's scoliosis screening program and furnish appropriate referral documents for parents.

An explanation of the benefits of the school district's screening program and all the forms necessary to carry it out are included. Specific instructions are given when necessary.

In some school districts, volunteers perform scoliosis screening. Other districts have the school nurse do the screening, while in larger districts, a small group of nurses or nurse practitioners may be selected to screen students.

FOLLOW-UP REPORT ON REFERRALS

The Follow-up Report on Referrals lists all referrals from a single campus to physicians. The form should be submitted to a designated authority (nurse supervisor or other administrator) within 30 days after the final screening on that campus. Be sure to include the parents' name, address, and home/work telephone numbers for those students with incomplete follow-up information.

SCOLIOSIS SCREENING: ANNUAL TOTALS BY CAMPUS

The Scoliosis Screening: Annual Totals by Campus lists all students screened for scoliosis. In a well-run scoliosis screening program, the physician referral rate, after rescreening, usually is about 3 to 5 percent of all children screened.

This form is followed by a filled-in sample. Here is an explanation of the symbols used in that sample:

1. John Jones is normal. He will not be rescreened.
2. Sally Smith has a right thoracic curve. She was rescreened two weeks later and referred to an orthopedist.
3. Andy Brown has a left lumbar curve so pronounced that he was referred without rescreening.
4. Sue Perez has a questionable left lumbar curve and still appears questionable a few days later. She will be rescreened in one year.
5. Rudy Garza has a left thoracic curve, but was normal on the two-week rescreen.

SCOLIOSIS SCREENING—ANNUAL TOTALS DISTRICTWIDE

The "Scoliosis Screening: Annual Totals Districtwide" is helpful for larger school districts with an organized scoliosis screening program. After diagnosis and referral, the school nurse can be most helpful in follow-up, probably the most difficult and time-consuming part of the entire program.

SCOLIOSIS SCREENING PROGRAM—PARENTAL NOTIFICATION

Dear Parents:

This year the _____ School District will be conducting a screening program to find children with scoliosis, or curvature of the spine. Similar screening programs in other states have shown that 7 to 10 children in every 100 may develop scoliosis and 1 to 3 will require treaatment. With early detection, through screening programs, severe spine deformity can be prevented.

The screening is carried out by the school nurse (practitioner). It is simple and takes less than 30 seconds per child. The examiner looks at the child's back and he or she stands and bends forward. If your child is found to have a possible curvature, you will be notified.

_____ School is scheduled to have its students evaluated the week of _____.

If, for any reason, you do not want your child to participate in the screening program, please notify the school principal.

SCOLIOSIS SCREENING PROGRAM—EXPLANATION FOR SCHOOL NURSE

I. Introduction

Scoliosis, a lateral curvature of the spine, is a relatively rare disorder that generally occurs in young adolescents. It is more common in girls than in boys.

Early detection is essential to achieve ideal treatment. The school provides an excellent setting in which to perform mass screening of the critical age groups. Screening will be carried out in the middle schools or high schools during P.E. classes when the students are dressed in gym clothes or bathing suits.

During the initial screening 5 to 10 percent of the students screened may be identified as possibly having curvature of the spine and require rescreening. Approximately two weeks after the initial screening, the nurse practitioners will return to the school campus to rescreen those students with questionable results. Three to 5 percent of those students who are rescreened usually require referral to a physician for further evaluation.

II. Program Goals

A. To identify students who may have scoliosis.
B. To provide students with factual information concerning scoliosis.
C. To provide an awareness of the implications of scoliosis for school personnel and for student's family.

III. Guidelines for Scoliosis Screening Program

The campus nurse will
1. Confirm with principal the date of screening.
2. Notify P.E. teachers of scoliosis screening date and arrange time to show film.
3. Prepare and send Notice of Scoliosis Screening form to parents of ____ and ____ grade students and students requiring reevaluation prior to scheduled day. Copies of notice for duplication on individual campuses are available from Health Services, Central Office. It is not necessary for students to return form to school.

PARENTAL NOTIFICATION OF SCOLIOSIS SCREENING RESULTS

Dear Parents,

During the recent scoliosis screening examination at school, your child was found to have physical signs of scoliosis. To rule out or confirm the presence of a spinal curvature, it is necessary to have an X ray or further examination by an orthopedic specialist.

To assist you in finding physicians that are experts in the diagnosis of spinal problems, we have enclosed a list of community resources that will provide examination and/or X ray at a reasonable charge. If you have a family physician, you may prefer to seek his recommendations.

Please complete the information below and return it to the school nurse so that clinics and physicians can plan for adequate time to examine students referred from the school. If you would like further information, please call your school nurse.

Sincerely,

---Tear Off Here---

1. I plan to make an appointment with _____for

   Name of doctor or clinic

   my child _____ to have further evaluation of a

   Name

   possible spine problem detected by the school screening program.

2. I would like further information regarding the dates reserved for _____ students.

   School _____

PARENTAL NOTIFICATION OF NORMAL SCREENING RESULTS

Dear Parents:

The X ray taken of your child's spine, as part of the school's scoliosis screening program, indicates that he or she does *not* have a spinal deformity.

No further treatment is recommended at this time. You are, however, encouraged to seek a reevaluation if there is any noticeable change in your child's posture.

Sincerely,

NOTIFICATION TO PARENT AND PHYSICIAN REGARDING
SCOLIOSIS SCREENING PROGRAM RESULTS

Name of student _____ **School** _____ **Grade** _____ **Date** _____

Dear Parents:

We have recently completed a screening for spinal deformity at your child's school. The test indicated that your child may have a possible curvature of the spine. The screening did not reveal the extent of the difficulty. It is urged that you contact your family physician or a pediatrician for further examination and advice. They may refer your child to an orthopedic surgeon for evaluation and treatment. If you do not have a family doctor or pediatrician, your school nurse will help you. Feel free to call.

Please take this sheet with you to your physician when your child is being examined and after examination return it to your school nurse.

Sincerely,

_____
Examiner

Dear Doctor:

The above child has been found to have some abnormal findings in a school Scoliosis Screening Program. Could you please review the findings? If your examination concurs and if indicated, a single *standing* posteroanterior X ray of the spine (film to include entire spine from shoulder to pubis) is suggested. The child must be standing with knees straight and not in a slouched posture. We request that you complete the following information so that we may continue to evaluate the screening program.

Physical exam shows:

X rays show:

Treatment or disposition:

Printed name _____
                                  Physician

Signature _____
                                  Physician

Instructions: Please return this entire page to school nurse.

SCOLIOSIS SCREENING
INDIVIDUAL REPORT

Patient no. _____

Name _____ D.O.B. _____ Sex: M _____ F _____

Parents _____ Address _____

School _____ Grade _____ Family physician _____

County _____ School year _____ Ethnic background: (1) Mexican-American _____ (4) Indian _____

(2) Caucasian _____ (5) Oriental _____

(3) Black _____ (6) Other _____

☐ New ☐ Follow-up

Report submitted by _____

History

Failure reasons, symptoms, complaints _____

_____

Prior awareness: No _____ Yes _____ How long: _____

Family history of scoliosis including relationships: No _____ Yes _____ _____

_____

Remarks _____

Under care   Other reason X ray

X ray refused _____ Prior to screening _____ Not taken _____

Screening X-ray Report

X ray taken at _____ Read by _____

X ray results: ☐ Negative   ☐ Scoliosis   ☐ Kyphosis/Lordosis   ☐ Other

Degree of scoliotic curve	Type of curve	Remarks
_____ Less than 10°	_____ Thoracic	
_____ 10° to 20°	_____ Double major	
_____ 20° to 40°	_____ Thoracolumbar	
_____ 40° to 55°	_____ Lumbar	
_____ More than 55°	_____ Other	

Recommendations

Discharge _____   Rescreen next year _____

Repeat AP standing X ray: 6 mos. _____   12 mos. _____   Other _____

Refer for orthopedic evaluation _____   Other _____

_____   _____

Date   Physician's signature

DOCTOR'S REPORT FOLLOWING SCOLIOSIS SCREENING

School _____

Teacher _____ Grade _____

Diagnosis _____

Treatment needed: _____ No _____ Yes _____

_____

Recommendations _____

_____

_____   _____   _____
          Child's name   Date   Doctor's signature

                                                              _____
                                                                        Address

                                                              _____
                                                                       Telephone

_____

I authorize the above information to be released to the _____ School District.

Date _____   Parent's signature _____

SCOLIOSIS SCREENING REFERRAL FORM—SECOND NOTICE

Name of student _____ **Date of birth** _____

School _____ **Grade** _____ **Date** _____

Dear Parents:

We recently completed a screening for spinal deformity at your child's school. The test indicated that your child may have a possible curvature of the spine, and we sent a referral notice urging you to contact your family physician or a pediatrician for further examination and advice. While updating our records, we find that we have received no response from you concerning your child.

Because curvature of the spine often gets worse, we urge you to have your child checked as soon as possible if you have not already done so. If your child has been examined, please send us the doctor's report.

To give you a better picture of what we saw on looking at your child's back, please note the diagrams below. You may note a similar curve of your child's back.

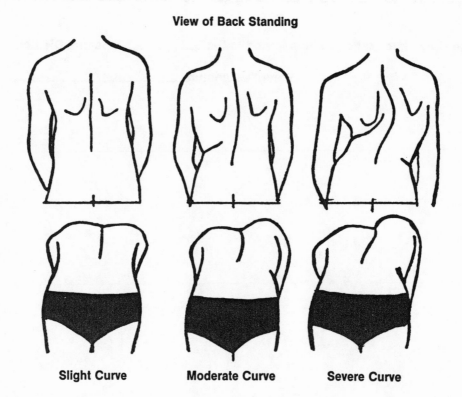

View of Back Standing

| Slight Curve | Moderate Curve | Severe Curve |

Please take the referral form with you when you see a physician. Return the completed form to the school nurse. Please call the school nurse if you have any questions or need help in making an appointment.

_____

School nurse

248

FOLLOW-UP REPORT ON SCOLIOSIS REFERRALS

Campus nurse _____   School _____

Name	Grade	Rm	D.O.B.	Date of assessment	Medical problem referred	Physician's diagnosis and recommendation	Date	Parent's name, address work/home telephone
1.								
2.								
3.								
4.								
5.								
6.								
7.								
8.								

SCOLIOSIS SCREENING: ANNUAL TOTALS BY CAMPUS

School _____ Grade _____

Name		Initial screen date						Rescreening date			
Last	First	H o m e r o o m	A g e	Results of bending test		R e s c r e e n	R e f e r	N e g a t i v e	R e f e r	R e s c r e e n 1 yr.	Comments
				Neg.	Pos. (list prob. area)						

Screeners _____

_____

R, right; L, left; T, thoracic; L, lumbar.

SCOLIOSIS SCREENING: ANNUAL TOTALS BY CAMPUS
(Filled-in sample)

School _____ Grade _____

Name		Initial screen date						Rescreening date			Comments
Last	First	Homeroom	Age	Results of bending test		Rescreen	Refer	Negative	Refer	Rescreen 1 yr	
				Neg.	Pos. (list prob. area)						
1. Jones, John		306	11	✓							
2. Smith, Sally		214	13		RT	✓			✓		
3. Brown, Andy		107	13		LL		✓				
4. Perez, Sue		116	12		LL?	✓				✓	
5. Garza, Rudy		107	13		LT	✓		✓			

Screeners _____

_____

R, right; L, left; T, thoracic; L, lumbar.

SCOLIOSIS SCREENING: ANNUAL TOTALS DISTRICTWIDE

School/Grade	Date screened	Enrollment	Number screened	Number refused screening	Number rescreened	Number referred	Students referred who						
							Were seen by physician	Did not require treatment or observation	Required observation by physician	Required brace	Required surgery	Required other treatment	Did not see a physician or no information available
Total													

FORMS FOR SPECIAL EDUCATION LIAISON

Almost all special education services are governed by federal and/or state legislation. While the federal guidelines are relatively uniform, the state guidelines vary.

Presented as examples, the forms in this section must be adapted to comply with each state's guidelines.

REQUEST FOR PSYCHIATRIC CONSULTATION

The Request for Psychiatric Consultation is a request from special education personnel to health services to provide contracted psychiatric services for an individual student.

HEALTH INFORMATION

The Health Information should be completed by the school nurse to accompany and complete the nursing assessment.

CONNORS' ABBREVIATED TEACHER'S SCHOOL REPORT

The Conners' Abbreviated Teacher's School Report helps to determine if medication is needed for hyperactivity and/or short attention span. The report should be initiated by the appropriate health professional and delivered to the appropriate classroom teacher. The teacher should observe the student in an academic setting, such as math or language arts. The comments section on this report can be used by the appropriate health professional and/or classroom teacher. Remarks should be limited to an objective explanation of observed behavior(s). The form should be returned to the appropriate health professional as soon as possible for appropriate follow-up.

ACTeRS PROFILE FOR BOYS

The ACTeRS PROFILE was recently developed by Dr. Rena Ullman and coworkers at the Institute for Child Behavior and Development at the University of Illinois at Urbana-Champaign. This sheet represents a sample filled out before and after the best dose of medication. The results are shown on the graph.

The ratings after Best Dose are shown for illustration only. In actual use, a separate sheet is used after each medication. "Best Dose" refers to that dose of medication that best controls the student's behavior without untoward side effects.

For example, the usual dose of Ritalin™ is $\frac{1}{10}$ to $\frac{1}{2}$ mgm per pound of body weight as a total daily dose. A 50-pound boy might start medication at about 5 to 10 mg a day, given 2.5 to 5 mg twice a day (in the morning and at noon) on school days. Since response to Ritalin™ is variable, the dose should be raised or lowered every three to five days until the "best" dose is reached.

HEALTH MANAGEMENT PLAN

The health component of the Individualized Education Plan (IEP) is to be completed on special education students with significant health problems.

For the following Health Management Plan,

1. List *only* "Findings" (signs, symptom, problems) that may require some action at school.
2. "Plan of Action" must contain a verb (administer, assist, develop, etc.) and clearly describe an activity that relates to the "Findings."
3. More than one person may be listed in the "Who/When" column, such as the teacher aide or nurse may participate in toileting activities. "When" may be simple: state "daily" or a specific date where appropriate.

SUGGESTIONS FOR HEALTH-RELATED SERVICES

The Suggestions for Health-Related Services differs from the usual IEP health component form. It may be used as a worksheet or as a final form to be inserted into the special education folder.

This format allows the health professional to describe the required related services in more detail.

ASSESSMENT DATA, ELIGIBILITY REPORTS

The purpose of these forms is to document a specific student's eligibility for a particular special education category when physician/nursing input is required.

Federal regulations list specific categories of special education. Most states require certain information to be supplied by various types of health professionals; however, each school district is allowed to develop its own forms—provided that all required information is supplied.

This information is often obtained directly from the physician. However, if school district policy permits, the school nurse may obtain the information by telephone, record it, sign the physician's name, and place his or her initials below, as is done in hospitals.

INDIVIDUAL ASSESSMENT: NOTICE AND CONSENT
(English)

Instructions: To be completed in conference with parent/guardian.

Student's name	Date of birth	School

The following kinds of tests may be used to find out more about how the student learns. Any or all of these tests will be used as needed. The results of the assessment will be used to assist school district personnel to develop an educational plan for the student.

Assessment Information

Type of information or test	Purpose
_____ Language	To see what language the student speaks and understands best.
_____ Speech	To find out how well the student can speak.
_____ Physical (may include general, medical, neurological, vision, and/or hearing)	To see if any physical problems affect the student's learning.
_____ Emotional/behavioral	To learn if the student has emotional or behavioral factors that may keep him from learning.
_____ Intellectual (verbal, nonverbal, adaptive)	To measure, in the student's own language or way of communicating, how well the student can understand, think and act over a wide range of experiences.
_____ Achievement tests	To see how well the student has learned in different subjects.
_____ Vocational assessments	To find out the student's vocational interest and attitude.

Notification of Procedural Safeguards

I understand my rights as the parent of a child with special needs and have received a copy of *Parent and Student Rights for a Special Education* (English/Spanish version.)

_____

Signature of parent/guardian (specify)

Parental Permission for Evaluation

_____ I give my permission for the personnel of the school district to evaluate my child at the school and/or Diagnostic Center.

If I am not able to accompany my child to the Diagnostic Center, permission is granted for district personnel to provide transportation.

_____ I do *not* give permission for my child to be evaluated.

Date	Signature of parent/guardian (specify)

EVALUACION INDIVIDUAL—AVISO Y CONSENTIMIENTO
(Spanish)

Instruciones: Para firmar en conferencia con el padre o guardian.

_____   _____   _____
Nombre del estudiante   Fecha de nacimiento   Escuela

Los siguientes tipos de pruebas pueden utilizarse para determinar el medio de aprendizaje del estudiante. Cualquiera de estas, o todas estas, pruebas se usarán segun se necesiten. Los resultados de la evaluación le servirán al personal del distrito escolar para desarrollar un plan educacional para el estudiante.

Evaluacion

Tipo de informacion o prueba

Proposito

_____ **Lenguaje**

Para determinar el lenguaje que el estudiante habla y entiende mejor.

_____ **Articulación**

Para determinar que tan bien habla el estudiante.

_____ **Fisico (puede incluir médico, neurológico, visual y, o, auditivo)**

Para determinar si algún problema fisico afecta el aprendizaje del estudiante.

_____ **Emocional/conducta**

Para determinar si existe algún factor emocional o de conducta que impida al estudiante aprender.

_____ **Intelectual (verbal, no verbal, o adaptivo)**

Para determinar, en el propio lenguaje o modo de comunicación del estudiante, que tan bien comprende, piensa, y actua sobre una variedad de experiencias.

_____ **Desempeño académico**

Para determinar que tan bien ha aprendido el estudiante en las diferentes materias.

_____ **Desempeño vocacional**

Para determinár el interes y la aptitud vocacional del estudiante.

Procedimiento para Protejer Sus Derechos

Yo entiendo mis derechos como padre de un (hijo) (hija) con necesidades especiales, y he recibido una copia de *Los Derechos de los Padres y Estudiantes a una Educación Especial* (versión en Ingles/Español)

_____
Firma del padre o guardian   (Especifique)

Permiso del Padre para la Evaluacion

_____ **Yo doy permiso para que el personal del Distrito Escolar Independiente de avalue a mi hijo/hija en la escuela y, o en el Centro Diagnostico.**

Si no me es pósible acompañar a mi hijo/hija al Centro Diagnóstico, doy permiso para que el personal del distrito (lo) (la) transporten.

_____ **No doy permiso para que mi (hijo) (hija) sea evaluado.**

_____   _____
Fecha   Firma del padre o guardian (Especifique)

LETTER OF NOTICE FROM
SPECIAL EDUCATION ASSESSMENT SERVICES

Date _____

To the parent of _____ Date of birth _____

Address _____ Grade _____

The Evaluation Committee of _____ School has requested an individual study of your child. The purpose of this study is to collect information that will help to better evaluate your child's educational needs and to plan a program to meet those needs.

To meet this request, we need your consent to the individual evaluation procedures that are described on the form that accompanies this letter. In the space provided below, the description of the evaluation procedures, please indicate your decision regarding the evaluation.

As the student's parent/legal guardian, you have the right to

> Refuse to permit evaluations or changes in your child's educational placement.
> Review all of your child's records.
> Review all tests and evaluation procedures.
> Be fully informed of the results of evaluations of your child.
> Give prior consent to or deny the disclosure of your child's school records to anyone other than school personnel.

In addition, following our evaluation and recommendations, you have the right to

> Request an independent evaluation, in accordance with federal guidelines and as specified in the booklet, *Parents and Students Rights for Special Education.*
> Request an impartial due process hearing if you wish to appeal any recommendations regarding your child's program.

You will be notified following the completion of your child's evaluation and will be invited to a meeting to discuss the results. At that time, any recommended changes in your child's program and/or special education placement will be reviewed. No changes will be made in your child's school program without your written permission.

If you have any questions or concerns, please call _____ at

_____.

_____

_____

_____

LETTER OF NOTICE FROM
SPECIAL EDUCATION ASSESSMENT SERVICES
Page 2

Student's name _____ Date received _____
             Last   **First**   **Middle**   **Month**   **Day**   **Year**

Birthdate _____ School _____

Student identification # _____ Student services # _____

_____

The evaluation procedures to be used for _____ (Name)
will cover the following areas:

Language:

Physical:

Emotional/behavioral:

Intellectual:

Sociological:

Communication:

(Please read attached explanation of tests.)

_____

I have been informed of the referral of my child, _____,
for individual testing or other evaluation procedures indicated above. I have received a copy of
Explanation of Procedural Safeguards and Due Process and understand my rights.

_____ I give my consent to conduct the evaluation described.

_____ I request a conference to discuss the referral of my child.

_____ I request a conference to discuss my rights as outlined in the enclosed information.

_____ I do not want my child evaluated at this time.

Date _____ _____
     Month   **Day**   **Year**   **Parent/legal guardian signature**

REQUEST FOR PSYCHIATRIC CONSULTATION

Date _____ School _____ Requested by _____ Student's name _____ D.O.B. _____

Principal's approval _____ Special Ed. category _____ Med/psychiatric diagnosis _____

Parent's name _____ Date of permission _____ N.P. _____

Medical

Summary and current status of any pertinent medical findings, tests reports, prenatal and developmental history, current and past medications (include dosage, who prescribed, date), results of prior consultations, and medical care including names of doctors and agencies.

Family Data

Family composition, any recent significant events, family history of mental or emotional disorder.

School

Specific concerns regarding behavior, academic level, instructional arrangement; describe time of day and context when behavior problem occurs; describe any time periods during the day when student is mainstreamed or unsupervised.

Summary of Test Data

Include any significant findings from assessment report.

PERMISSION FORM FOR PSYCHIATRIC CONSULTATION

Name_____Birthdate_____School_____

Please list all prescription medications that your child is taking:

Medicine	Dose	Time of day taken	Given by home or school?	For what problem?

Other comments:

Is your child under the care of a doctor? _____ Yes   _____ No

If yes, may we contact the doctor about your child? _____ Yes   _____ No

Name and agency or address of doctor _____
                                    Name   **Agency or address**

I give permission for my child to be interviewed at school by school district physicians or consultants. If medicine is needed to help my child to learn at school, I give permission for the medicine to be prescribed, and I will help to see that it is given. I understand that there will be no charge for the psychiatric consultation, but I will be expected to purchase any necessary medication. I understand that I will be contacted by the physician or nurse practitioner before the medicine is prescribed or changed. I understand that I will be notified of my child's appointment with the doctor, and I will attempt to be present at the school for that appointment.

_____   _____
        Date   **Parent's signature**

HEALTH INFORMATION

Student's name _____ Birthdate _____
                                                                    Mo.   Day   Yr.

Student's identification no. _____ Student services no. _____

School _____ Grade _____ Section _____

Vision: R _____ L _____ Date tested _____ Comment/type test _____
                                          Mo.   Day   Yr.

Hirschberg   **Color Vision**   **Plus Lens**

Hearing: R _____ L _____ Date tested _____ Comment/type test _____
                                            Mo.   Day   Yr.

Brief health history: Date _____ Informant _____

☐ **New referral**   ☐ **Current medical exam available**

☐ **Reevaluation**   Date of exam/examiner

☐   ☐ **Nurse to participate in IEP**   ☐ **Medical pending; appt. date** _____
Yes No

                                         ☐ **Medical examination not indicated**

                                         ☐ **Specialty examination needed/available** _____
                                                                                        Type

                                    _____ Date _____
                                         School nurse

REQUEST FOR NURSING ASSESSMENT

Name _____ _____ _____
  Last   First   M   Student I.D. No.   D.O.B.

_____
School

Instructions: This page may be detached for completion by or use of the nurse and/or physician. Consult with nurse for educational implications of any abnormalities (e.g., seat placement for vision or hearing loss).

1. **Vision screening**   Date _____

   Without glasses: R _____ L _____

   With glasses: R _____ L _____

   Interpretation

After 5th birthday:		20/40	**Abnormal**
		20/30	**Normal**
Before fifth birthday:		20/50	**Abnormal**
		20/40	**Normal**

2. **Hearing screening**
   Tympanometric screening

   Initial Date   **Retest Date (if required)**
   Normal   ☐   **Normal**   ☐
   Abnormal ☐   **Abnormal** ☐
   or
   Audiometric screening Date _____
   Normal   ☐
   Abnormal ☐
   (Graph for abnormal only)

   Interpretation

25–40	**Mild**	70–90	**Severe**
40–55	**Marginal**	90+	**Profound**
55–70	**Moderate**		

   Audiogram

   .10
   0
   10
   20
   30
   40
   50
   60
   70
   80
   90
   100
        500   1000   2000   4000
   Speech   **Range**
   O (Right)   **X (Left)**

3. **Physical assessment/examination: Date performed** _____

   Height _____ Weight _____ Head circumference _____ Blood pressure _____

   Abnormal findings (Do not leave blank if assessment is normal. Write "None.") _____

   _____

   _____

4. **Is this student on medication? Yes** _____ **No** _____ **If yes** _____

   Given at: Home _____ **School** _____ **Both** _____

5. **Additional remarks concerning health status** _____

   _____

   _____

Date _____ Physician/nurse _____

SCHOOL HEALTH ASSESSMENT SUMMARY

Student _____ Birthdate _____

School _____ Grade _____

Review of School Health Records
(Record any past medical problems that are of significance):
     Chronic health problem(s):

     Significant health history from original assessment:

     Significant health history since last staffing:

Current Findings or Concerns
(Record current health history and assessment information):

     Vision _____ Date _____ Hearing _____ Date _____

     Height _____ Percentile _____ Weight _____ Percentile _____

     Current medications:

Current health status (Include chronic as well as acute):

Nursing Comments
(State present level of physical functioning in educator term):

Recommendations
(List health needs in educator terms):

Date _____ School nurse _____

HOME/HOSPITAL BOUND PROGRAM—SCHOOL REFERRAL

Instructions: Please print or type. Return original and duplicates.

_____/ _____/ _____ _____ _____
Student's name, Last   **First**   **Middle**   **Birthdate**   **Sex**

_____ **Home** _____ **Business** _____
Address of student   **Telephone**

_____ _____ _____ _____
          School   **Student identification number**   **Grade**   **Ethnic group**
                                            (name is)

Student lives with _____ **whose (names are)** _____

Student is expected to be confined at home/hospital for _____ **weeks because of** _____

The program of Home/Hospital Bound teaching is closely coordinated with the school to which a student is expected to return.

Cooperating teachers are assigned to work with the home/hospital teacher who serves as liaison between school and home/hospital.

All procedures, including the selection of courses and planning of the schedule for permanently homebound students unable to take a full course of study leading to accumulation of credits, will be directed by the Special Education Department in cooperation with the principal of the home school in proportion to the physical and mental abilities of the individual.

As recommended by the physician, this student will participate in a modified health program or one of complete rest and will receive Physical Education credit each quarter under the direction of the home/hospital teacher. This is in accord with the policy.

During the period of Home/Hospital Bound instruction, attendance and grades will be reported by the home/hospital teacher to the student's home school, where all records will be kept.

Class period	Subjects	Cooperating teacher	Room	Grades for current year								
				1st	2nd	Cr.	3rd	4th	Cr.	5th	6th	Cr.

_____   _____
        Date   **Signature of principal or guidance counselor**

HOME/HOSPITAL BOUND PROGRAM—STATEMENT
OF PARENT/GUARDIAN

Instructions: Please print or type. Return original and duplicates.

_____/ _____/ _____ _____
Student's name, Last   First   Middle   Birthdate

                                                                    Home   **Business**
_____ _____
Address of student   Telephone

_____ _____ _____
        School   Grade   Hospital

_____ _____ _____
        Name of physician   Address of physician   Telephone

Teaching under the Home/Hospital Bound Program is requested for the above-named student.

A proper setting for learning will be provided that includes a responsible adult in the home but not in the room.

The place provided will be clean, well lighted, quiet, free from disturbances, and properly heated and ventilated.

Working space and furniture adjustments will be made in accordance with the physician's recommendations for the student during the time he or she is doing his school work.

Changes in the home teaching program may be necessary from time to time as other students are added to or dropped from the teacher's roll; as a result, I understand that my child's schedule will have to be adjusted accordingly.

I shall notify the home/hospital teacher, if my child is ill or unable to have his lesson.

It is my understanding that home/hospital teaching cannot begin until the above conditions have been met and that home/hospital teaching will be discontinued if these conditions are not maintained.

I understand that the student's educational program will be planned and carried out on the basis of the limitations of the student. I authorize the referring physician to release available medical information requested _____ for this purpose.

┌─────────────────────────────────┐
│ **Return to:**   │
│ **Special Education Office**   │
└─────────────────────────────────┘
                                          _____
                                          Signature of parent/guardian

                                          _____
                                                        Date

_____
Date received in Special Education Office

267

HOME/HOSPITAL BOUND PROGRAM—STATEMENT OF PHYSICIAN

Instructions: Please check statement carefully and fill in all blanks to prevent delay in planning student's program. Return original and duplicates.

_____/_____/_____ _____
Student's name, Last   First   Middle   Birthdate

_____ _____
                              Student's address   Home
                                                                                                   Telephone

For _____ weeks the above-named student will be unable to attend a regular school or special class. (Physician must anticipate that the student will be absent for at least _____ weeks.)

This student needs to continue school work at home or in the hospital under the Home/Hospital Bound Program, and this work will not interfere with recovery.

The student's illness (is) (is not) communicable, infectious, or contagious to others at this time.

Diagnosis of the student's illness is as follows: _____

_____

Are there other health problems?   ☐ Yes   ☐ No

If "yes," explain. _____

_____

Are there vision or hearing problems suspected?   ☐ Yes   ☐ No

If "yes," explain. _____

Restrictions that the home/hospital teacher should observe in working with the student are as follows:

    1. Length of time for activity _____

    2. Position: Flat _____. Upright _____. _____

    3. Length of sitting time _____

Precautions are _____

_____

Prognosis for improvement is_____ Prognosis for life is_____

Return to:
Special Education Office

_____
Date received in Special Education Office

_____
Signature of physician

_____
Printed name of physician

_____
Date

_____
Address of physician

_____
Office telephone

HOME/HOSPITAL BOUND PROGRAM—PHYSICIAN CLEARANCE
TO RETURN TO SCHOOL

Instructions: Please return original and duplicate.

_____/ _____/ _____ _____

Student's name, Last   First   Middle   Birthdate

_____ _____ _____

          Student's address   **Home**   **Business**

          Student's address   Telephone

_____ _____

          School   Grade

The above-named student may return to school on _____

                                                   Date

following an illness or incapacity of the following nature: _____

_____

_____

Limitation of activities are as follows. (Please state the length of time these limitations are to be observed.)

_____

_____

_____

Other instructions regarding care of the student at school _____

_____

_____

This completed form should accompany the student upon returning to school from the Home/Hospital Bound Program.	_____ Signature of physician _____ Printed name of physician _____ Date _____ Address of physician _____ Office telephone

CONNERS' ABBREVIATED TEACHER'S SCHOOL REPORT

Date _____

Student services # _____

Name _____ School _____

Ethnic group or race _____ Grade _____ Birthdate _____

Instructions: Check the appropriate box for each item, not at all, just a little, pretty much *or* very much, *that best describes your assessment of the child. Please complete all ten items.*

Observation	Degree of Activity			
	0 Not at all	1 Just a little	2 Pretty much	3 Very much
1. Restless or overactive				
2. Excitable, impulsive				
3. Disturbs other children				
4. Fails to finish things he/she starts, short attention span				
5. Constantly fidgeting				
6. Inattentive, easily distracted (interferes with learning)				
7. Demands must be met immediately, is easily frustrated				
8. Cries often and easily				
9. Mood changes quickly and drastically				
10. Temper outbursts, explosive and unpredictable behavior				

Initiated by _____   _____
              Health professional   Observer's signature

Comments:
                                                                          A.M.
_____   _____ P.M.
            Area of instruction   Time of day

ADD COMPREHENSIVE TEACHER'S RATING SCALE (ACTeRS)

Before medication ☐   After medication ☐

Instructions: To be completed by classroom teacher. Below are descriptions of children's behavior. Please read each item and compare this child's behavior to his or her classmates. Circle the number that most closely corresponds with your evaluation. Return to campus nurse.

Child's name _____   School _____

Rater _____   Date _____ Grade _____

	Almost never				Almost always	
Behavior item						
Works well independently	1	2	3	4	5	
Persists with task for reasonable amount of time	1	2	3	4	5	
Completes assigned tasks satisfactorily with little additional assistance	1	2	3	4	5	**Attention**
Follows simple directions accurately	1	2	3	4	5	
Follows a sequence of instructions	1	2	3	4	5	
Functions well in the classroom	1	2	3	4	5	
Add all numbers circled and place total here						Score _____
Extremely overactive (out of seat, "on the go")	1	2	3	4	5	
Overreacts	1	2	3	4	5	**Hyperactivity**
Fidgety (hands always busy)	1	2	3	4	5	
Impulsive (acts or talks without thinking)	1	2	3	4	5	
Restless (squirms in seat)	1	2	3	4	5	
Add all numbers circled and place total here						Score _____
Behaves positively with peers/classmates	1	2	3	4	5	
Verbal communication clear and connected	1	2	3	4	5	**Social Skills**
Nonverbal communication accurate	1	2	3	4	5	
Follows group norms and special rules	1	2	3	4	5	
Cites general rule when criticizing ("We aren't supposed to do that . . .")	1	2	3	4	5	
Skillful at making new friends	1	2	3	4	5	
Approaches new situations confidently	1	2	3	4	5	
Add all numbers circled and place total here						Score _____
Tries to get others into trouble	1	2	3	4	5	
Starts fights over nothing	1	2	3	4	5	**Oppositional**
Makes malicious fun of others	1	2	3	4	5	
Defies authority	1	2	3	4	5	
Picks on others	1	2	3	4	5	
Mean and cruel to other children	1	2	3	4	5	
Add all numbers circled and place total here						Score _____

Courtesy of Rina K. Ullmann, Robert L. S. Prague, and Esther K. Sleator, Institute for Child Behavior and Development, University of Illinois at Urbana. Reproduced by permission of copyright holder.

ADD COMPREHENSIVE TEACHER'S RATING SCALE (ACTeRS)
(Filled-in sample)

Instructions: To be completed by classroom teacher. Below are descriptions of children's behavior. Please read each item and compare this child's behavior to his or her classmates. Circle the number that most closely corresponds with your evaluation.

Child's name _____ School _____

Rater _____ Date _____ Grade _____

Behavior item	Almost never			Almost always			Ratings on best dose
Works well independently	①	2	3	4	5		
Persists with task for reasonable amount of time	①	2	3	4	5		
Completes assigned tasks satisfactorily with little additional assistance	①	2	3	4	5	Attention	
Follows simple directions accurately	1	②	3	4	5		
Follows a sequence of instructions	1	②	3	4	5		
Functions well in the classroom	①	2	3	4	5		
Add all numbers circled and place total here						Score _8_	25
Extremely overactive (out of seat, "on the go")	1	2	3	④	5		
Overreacts	1	2	3	④	5	Hyperactivity	
Fidgety (hands always busy)	1	2	3	④	5		
Impulsive (acts or talks without thinking)	1	2	3	④	5		
Restless, squirms in seat	1	2	3	④	5		
Add all numbers circled and place total here						Score 20	10
Behaves positively with peers/classmates	1	②	3	4	5		
Verbal communication clear and connected	1	2	3	4	⑤	Social skills	
Nonverbal communication accurate	1	2	3	④	5		
Follows group norms and special rules	1	②	3	4	5		
Cites general rule when criticizing ("We aren't supposed to do that . . .")	1	2	3	④	5		
Skillful at making new friends	1	②	3	4	5		
Approaches new situations confidently	1	②	3	4	5		
Add all numbers circled and place total here						Score 23	24
Tries to get others into trouble	1	②	3	4	5		
Starts fights over nothing	1	②	3	4	5	Oppositional	
Makes malicious fun of others	1	②	3	4	5		
Defies authority	1	②	3	4	5		
Picks on others	1	②	3	4	5		
Mean and cruel to other children	1	②	3	4	5		
Add all numbers circled and place total here						Score 12	9

BEHAVIORAL EVALUATION REPORT ACTeRS PROFILE

Name _____ D.O.B. _____

School _____ Grade _____ Date _____

Percentile	Attention	Hyperactivity	Social skills	Oppositional
95			35	
90			34	
80	30		33	
	29		32	
	28	5	31	
70	27	6	30	
	26	7		
	25		29	
		8		
60	24		28	
		9		
	23		27	
50		10		6
	22	11	26	7
	21		25	
	20			8
40	19	12		9
		13	24	10
			23	11
		14		
	18			
30		15		12
			22	
	17			13
20	16	16	21	14
	15	17	20	15
	14	18	19	16
	13	19	18	18
10	12	20	17	19
5	11	21		20
		22	16	21 or more
		23	15 or less	
	6–10	24		

Instructions: Circle the raw scores from the teacher's rating scale in each of the four columns. Percentiles are shown in the leftmost column. Use blue pen to reflect scores obtained before medication; use red pen to reflect scores after medication.

Results:
  Below 20 percentile, abnormal
  20 to 40 percentile, moderate
  Above 40 percentile, normal

Comments _____

_____

_____

_____

_____

_____

273

BEHAVIORAL EVALUATION REPORT ACTeRS PROFILE
(Filled-in sample)

Name _____ D.O.B. _____

School _____ Grade _____ Date _____

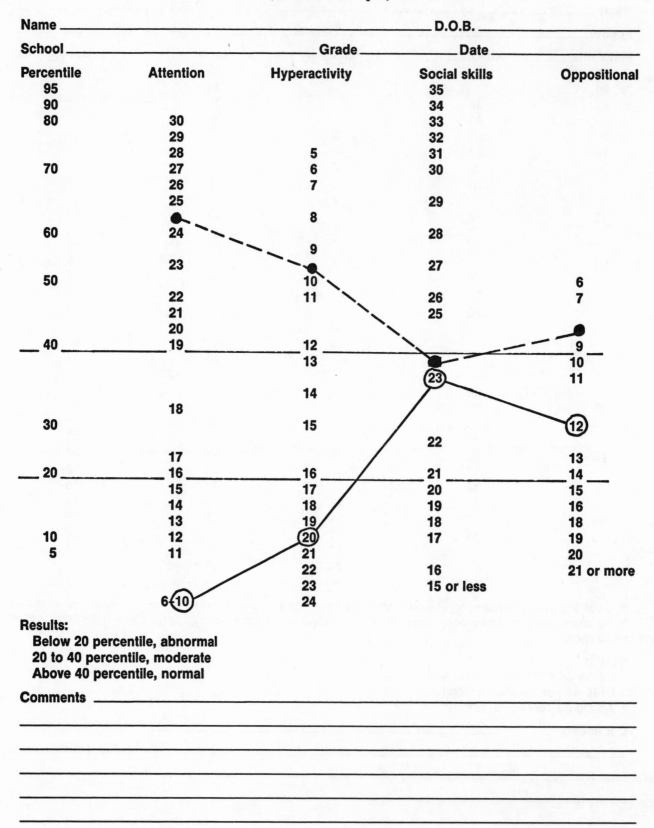

Results:
Below 20 percentile, abnormal
20 to 40 percentile, moderate
Above 40 percentile, normal

Comments _____

_____

_____

_____

_____

_____

INDIVIDUALIZED EDUCATION PROGRAM

Date _____ Review date _____

☐ Initial Ekg. Meeting _____

☐ Annual review _____

☐ Transfer review _____

☐ Triannial Reeval. _____

Original—Spec. Educ. Office
Copy—Parent
Copy—Spec. Educ. Teacher—DIS

Pupil _____

Address _____

Birthdate _____ Current grade _____ Sex _____

Current school _____ Current teacher _____

Special Education Program _____

Parent/guardian _____

Home phone _____ Work phone _____

Primary language of pupil _____ ☐ LES

Primary language of home _____ ☐ NES

Present levels of educational performance	Annual goals	Short-term objectives to include evaluation criteria	Person responsible	Evaluation
Reading				**Objective(s)** ☐ Met ☐ Drop ☐ See new IEP Date _____ Eval. by _____
Math				**Objective(s)** ☐ Met ☐ Drop ☐ See new IEP Date _____ Eval. by _____
Written language				**Objective(s)** ☐ Met ☐ Drop ☐ See new IEP Date _____ Eval. by _____
Health/medical				**Objective(s)** ☐ Met ☐ Drop ☐ See new IEP Date _____ Eval. by _____

INDIVIDUALIZED EDUCATION PROGRAM
(Filled-in sample)

Original—Spec. Educ. Office
Copy—Parent
Copy—Spec. Educ. Teacher—DIS

Date _1/20/87_   Review date _1/88_

☐ Initial Ekg. Meeting _____
☑ Annual review _____
☐ Transfer review _____
☐ Triannial Reeval. _____

Pupil _Kim Nguyen_

Address _7997 Broadway Apt. 6_

Birthdate _6/26/79_ Current grade _3_ Sex _F_

Current school _Taft_ Current teacher _Taylor_

Special Education Program _Resource Specialist Program_

Parent/guardian _Nguyen, Danh – Father_

Home phone _123-4567_ Work phone _765-4321_

Primary language of pupil _Vietnamese_ ☑ LES

Primary language of home _Vietnamese_ ☐ NES

Present levels of educational performance	Annual goals	Short-term objectives to include evaluation criteria	Person responsible	Evaluation
Reading 1/87 WRAT 25 – Word Recognition Brigance 2.2 – Word Recognition Primer – Oral Reading + Comprehension – Knows 87/250 Sight Words Knows 12/24 Ending Sounds Knows Short Vowels. 1/5 Long Vowels Knows 22/33 Initial Clusters Visually 0/33 " " Auditorily	To improve Reading Skills	Given a reading passage at the 1st grade level, Kim Nguyen will read fluently decode new words and answer comprehension questions with 80% accuracy as measured by teacher test Brigance or observation. Given 20 words with long vowels Kim will sound out words with 80% accuracy as measured by teacher test, Brigance or observation.	Classroom Teacher/ Resource Specialist	Objective(s) ☐ Met ☐ Drop ☐ See new IEP Date _____ Eval. by _____
Math 1/87 WRAT 35 Computation Skills Brigance 3.5 " " Knows Basic Addition + Subtraction Facts – Not Consistent with Regrouping in Addition + Subtraction	To continue current progress in math			Objective(s) ☐ Met ☐ Drop ☐ See new IEP Date _____ Eval. by _____
Written language 1/87 WRAT 2.2 Spelling Brigance – Could not do sentence dictation. Currently mastering 10 words a week at the Primer level. Can write upper + lower case letters sequentially. Can do 5/33 initial clusters dictated.	To improve written expression skills.	Given 20 words with initial clusters dictated, Kim will identify clusters with 80% accuracy as measured by Brigance teacher test or observation. Given a weekly list of spelling words at the 2nd grade level, Kim will spell words, when dictated, with 80% accuracy as measured by teacher test.	Classroom Teacher/ Resource Specialist	Objective(s) ☐ Met ☐ Drop ☐ See new IEP Date _____ Eval. by _____
Health/medical Seizure Disorder – Under medical supervision at Humana. Rx Tegretol 800 mg. Volproic Acid 500 mg. Daily. Still having seizures 1-5 times per week (lasting 1-3 min)	To follow medical recommendations to have a better understanding of seizure disorder	Given weekly health counseling sessions, Kim will have an understanding of the disease process by verbally describing what happens before during + after a seizure @ 70% accurate. She will improve self concept by better interpersonal relationship as justified by teachers and nurse.		Objective(s) ☐ Met ☐ Drop ☐ See new IEP Date _____ Eval. by _____

INDIVIDUALIZED EDUCATION PROGRAM DOCUMENT

I. Identification Information	II. Goal Statement Summary
Student name _____ Last First Middle **Date of birth** _____ **Teacher** _____ **School** _____ **Date of meeting** _____	**Annual goal:** _____ _____ _____

III. Short-Term Objectives Planning Section

Objectives	Criteria for review	Method/procedure of evaluation	Date of review
A.			
B.			
C.			
D.			

IV. Unit Review Section (Review of progress)

____ **Exceeded criteria** **A.** ____ **Met criteria** ____ **Did not meet criteria** **Date of review** _____ **Comments:**	____ **Exceeded criteria** **B.** ____ **Met criteria** ____ **Did not meet criteria** **Date of review** _____ **Comments:**	____ **Exceeded criteria** **C.** ____ **Met criteria** ____ **Did not meet criteria** **Date of review** _____ **Comments:**	____ **Exceeded criteria** **D.** ____ **Met criteria** ____ **Did not meet criteria** **Date of review** _____ **Comments:**

V. Goal Statement Annual Review

Review of student progress: ____ Exceeded criteria* ____ Met criteria ____ Did not meet criteria*

Recommendation: ____ No longer requires special assistance to meet this goal.   *Explain: _____

_____ Continue short-term objectives as described above.

_____ Modify short-term objectives.

_____ Develop alternative short-term objectives.

Comments:

_____

_____

_____

277

INDIVIDUALIZED EDUCATION PROGRAM DOCUMENT
(Filled-in sample)

I. Identification Information

Student name _DOE_ _MARY_ _X._
            Last   First   Middle

Date of birth _3-19-78_

Teacher _TAYLOR_   School _TAFT_

Date of meeting _JUNE 1987_

II. Goal Statement Summary

Annual goal: _To develop Self-Directed Management of Cerebral Palsy so that her participation in total program will increase._

III. Short-Term Objectives Planning Section

Objectives	Criteria for review	Method/procedure of evaluation	Date of review
A. Mary will take medication as prescribed for a two-month period.	Information obtained from student, parent, physician, will confirm.	1. Student log 2. Parental feedback 3. Telephone contacts with physician.	11/87
B. Mary will follow prescribed physical activity regimen 90% of the time for 4 months	Information obtained from student, parent, physician, physical therapist will confirm.	1. Behavioral Chart 2. Verbal feedback from student, parent, therapist	1/88
C. Mary will maintain prescribed regimen of rest.	Greater self-reliance in avoiding fatigue. Fewer absences.	1. Fewer self-initiated visits to school nurse 2. Improved attendance record	4/88
D. Mary will increase her participation in school, social and recreational activities by 50%.	Will participate at least 50% of the time.	1. Student log 2. Verbal feedback from parent, teacher, counselor. 3. School nurse observation	6/88

IV. Unit Review Section (Review of progress)

___ Exceeded criteria **A.**	___ Exceeded criteria **B.**	✓ Exceeded criteria **C.**	✓ Exceeded criteria **D.**
✓ Met criteria	___ Met criteria	___ Met criteria	___ Met criteria
___ Did not meet criteria	✓ Did not meet criteria	___ Did not meet criteria	___ Did not meet criteria
Date of review _8/15/87_	Date of review _10/15/87_	Date of review _10/15/87_	Date of review _10/15/87_
Comments:	Comments:	Comments:	Comments:

V. Goal Statement Annual Review

Review of student progress: ___ Exceeded criteria* ✓ Met criteria ___ Did not meet criteria*

Recommendation: ___ No longer requires special assistance to meet this goal.   *Explain: _____

        ___ Continue short-term objectives as described above.   _____

        ✓ Modify short-term objectives.   _____

        ___ Develop alternative short-term objectives.   _____

Comments:

HEALTH MANAGEMENT PLAN (IEP-RELATED SERVICES)

Student _____ D.O.B. _____ Completed by _____
　　　　　Last　　　　　　　　　　First

School _____ /Grade _____ I.D. no. _____ Adaptive no. _____ Date _____

Diagnosis/eligibility _____ Column II code _____

　　　　　_____ Update/review _____

Problems/concerns	Negative/Normal	Findings (signs/symptoms/problems)	Plan of action	Who/when
I. A. Medical				
B. Dental				
II. Medication				
III. Mobility/coordination				
A. Ambulation/ position				
B. Activities/ adaptive P.E.				
IV. Self-help				
A. Eating				
B. Oral hygiene				
C. Elimination				
D. Communication				
V. Other				

HEALTH MANAGEMENT PLAN (IEP-RELATED SERVICES)
(Filled-in sample)

Student _____ D.O.B. _6/19/76_   Completed by _____

      Last   First

School _J.N. BRYAN_ /Grade _4C_ I.D. no. _625510_ Adaptive no. ____   Date _9/87 UPDATE_

Diagnosis/eligibility _HEARING IMPAIRED - REQUIRING HEARING AID_   Column II code _A_

_____   Update/review _YEARLY_

Problems/concerns	Negative/Normal	Findings (signs/symptoms/problems)	Plan of action	Who/when
I. A. Medical		Hearing loss –severe requiring aid as evaluated @ Callier – 8/86 –	School RN– Conf. ē teacher –re: wearing of Aid & Aid maintenance	School RN/ teacher (beginning school yr.)
B. Dental				
II. Medication	✓		Refer for f/u – PRN as indicated (no apparent problems during summer– 1988	yrly. + PRN School/RN/teacher parent
III. Mobility/coordination	✓			
A. Ambulation/ position	✓			
B. Activities/ adaptive P.E.	✓			
IV. Self-help	✓			
A. Eating	✓			
B. Oral hygiene	✓			
C. Elimination	✓			
D. Communication		Speech problem	enrolled in speech therapy	speech clinician parent, teacher
V. Other				

SUGGESTIONS FOR HEALTH-RELATED SERVICES

Name _____ Date of birth _____

School _____ Grade _____ Date of IEP meeting _____

Instructions: To be used for special education students who require health-related services. To be completed by appropriate health services professional—school nurse, OT, PT, physician, etc.—to describe briefly which services are necessary. Other appropriate health-related items may be added in each category. Nurse practitioners, nursing supervisors, or school physician may be consulted if necessary. To be forwarded to Health Services office prior to IEP committee meeting for inclusion in IEP as deemed appropriate.

Medications: Name of medication, dosage and time of administration, significant adverse side effects, designation of individual plus an alternate to give it.

Braces, walkers, and other appliances: Type of appliance, care at school (need for removal, change, adjustment, etc.), instruction of personnel in student's use of appliance.

Medical procedures (catheterization, suction, ostomy bags, toileting, etc.): Equipment needed; catheter, flats, KY, etc., Who supplies equipment? Time of performance of procedure. Designated individual to perform?

Classroom seat location, free access, part-time attendance: Is special seat location necessary? If so, where? Are ramps or elevators necessary? Does medical condition limit full-day attendance?

Adaptation of P.E. program: Can child monitor own level of physical activity or should periods of rest be prescribed? If so, how much? Should any activities be restricted (e.g., swimming, weight lifting, running)?

Physical, occupational, orientation, therapy: Is it necessary? Who will perform it? How often? How much will parent/teacher/aide participate?

Liaison with attending physician: Are periodic reports necessary? If so, how often? Designation of personnel to report.

Other: Describe below.

_____

Brief listing only of those procedures or services necessary *during school day.*

Approved by _____

_____   _____
Signature   Title

_____   _____
Date   Location

PHYSICAL EXAMINATION PERMISSION FORM—
VOCATIONAL ADJUSTMENT PROGRAM

I. **Student's name** _____ **Date of birth** _____

   Room/teacher _____ **School** _____ **Date** _____

        I hereby give permission for my son/daughter _____
to receive a physical examination, at no cost to myself, for participation in the Vocational Adjustment
Program.

_____   _____

Date   **Signature of parent or guardian**

II. *Instructions: To be completed by school nurse.*   **Date** _____

   Height   _____   **Vision: With glasses**   RT 20/_____ L 20/_____

   Weight   _____   **Without glasses**   RT 20/_____ L 20/_____

   Pulse rate   _____   **Hearing (spoken voice)**   RT normal _____ abnormal_____

   Blood pressure _____   **L** normal _____ abnormal _____

   Condensed medical history _____

   _____

   _____

   Alleged handicap _____

   _____

   _____

III. *Instructions: To be completed by physician.*   **Date** _____

   **Physical examination code: O, satisfactory, 1X, slight; 2X, unsatisfactory; 3X, marked unsatisfactory;
OO, previous correction.**

          Nose   _____   **Lungs**   _____

          Teeth   _____   **Chest**   _____

          Tonsils _____   **Spine**   _____

          Ears   _____   **Hernia**   _____

          Heart   _____   **Genitalia** _____

   Physical capabilities code: √, no limitations; X, limitation; O, to be avoided.

          Pulling   _____   **Walking** _____

          Lifting   _____   **Stooping** _____

          Pushing _____   **Kneeling** _____

          Reaching _____   **Other**   _____

   Findings and/or impressions _____

   _____

_____   _____

Physician's printed name   **Physician's signature**

ASSESSMENT DATA, ELIGIBILITY REPORT: MENTALLY RETARDED

_____   _____   _____
Name of student   Chronological age   Date of birth

_____   _____
Name of school   Date of assessment

Professional evaluator: Licensed or certified psychologist, certified psychological associate, or educational diagnostician.

_____ (is/is not) functioning two or more standard deviations
Name of student   below the mean in

verbal ability, as measured by_____(_____) _____   ☐   ☐
                                              S.D.   Date   Yes   No

nonverbal or performance ability, as measured by_____(_____)_____   ☐   ☐
                                                    S.D.   Date   Yes   No

This student (appears, does not appear) to have a deficit in adaptive behavior as measured by_____

_____   _____
                                                     Date

_____ (does/does not) appear to meet specific eligibility
Name of student
criteria for mental retardation. Comments:

Degree of mental retardation (e.g., mild, moderate, severe, profound; I.Q. score):

Implications for student's education:

_____   _____   _____
Signature   Position   Date

ASSESSMENT DATA, ELIGIBILITY REPORT: EMOTIONALLY DISTURBED

_____   _____   _____
Name of student   **Chronological age**   **Date of birth**

_____   _____
Name of school   **Date of assessment**

Professional evaluator: Licensed or certified psychologist, psychological associate, psychiatrist.

Over a period of time and to a degree that adversely affects educational performance _____
                                                                     Name of student

does exhibit the following characteristics:

	Yes	**No**
An inability to learn that cannot be explained by intellectual, sensory, or health factors.	☐	☐
An inability to build or maintain satisfactory interpersonal relationships with peers and teacher.	☐	☐
Inappropriate types of behavior or feelings under normal circumstances.	☐	☐
A general pervasive mood of unhappiness or depression.	☐	☐
A tendency to develop physical symptoms or fears associated with personal or school problems.	☐	☐

Based on these factors, _____ **(does/does not) appear to meet**
                                 Name of student

eligibility criteria for emotional disturbance.

Type of emotional disturbance:

Severity of emotional disturbance:

Source(s) of data:

ASSESSMENT DATA, ELIGIBILITY REPORT: EMOTIONALLY DISTURBED
(Page 2)

Implications for student's education:

Degree to which this student's documented in-school and out-of-school behavior is consistent with (1) the diagnosis and (2) the identified behavior that is considered to be a direct result of the emotional handicap:

Recommendations for behavioral management in the educational setting:

_____	_____	_____
Signature	**Position**	**Date**
_____	_____	_____
(Signature of psychological associate supervisor. Must be licensed or certified psychologist.)	**Position**	**Date**

ASSESSMENT DATA, ELIGIBILITY REPORT: MULTIPLY HANDICAPPED

_____   _____   _____
Name of student   **Chronological age**   **Date of birth**

_____   _____
Name of school   **Date of report**

Professional evaluator(s): Licensed physician, psychiatrist, psychologist, psychological associate, educational diagnostician.

Written reports documenting eligibility criteria are attached for the following (two or more) handicapping conditions.

_____   _____
Handicapping condition   **Date of report**

These handicapping conditions are expected to continue indefinitely.   ☐   ☐
                                                                                   Yes   No

This student's disabilities do require comprehensive instruction and related services in programs for the severely handicapped.   ☐   ☐
                                                                                   Yes   No

The disabilities do impair performance in _all_ of the following areas: ☐   ☐
                                                                                   Yes   No

Area	**Documentation**
☐ **Psychomotor skills**	_____
☐ **Self-care skills**	_____
☐ **Communication skills**	_____
☐ **Social and emotional development**	_____
☐ **Cognition**	_____

_____ **(does/does not) appear to meet all of the**
Name of student
eligibility criteria

_____ **as a multiply handicapped student.**

_____ **implications for student's education.**

_____   _____   _____
Signature   **Position**   **Date**

_____   _____   _____
Signature   **Position**   **Date**

286

ASSESSMENT DATA, ELIGIBILITY REPORT: VISUALLY HANDICAPPED

Part I

_____   _____   _____
Name of student   **Chronological age**   **Date of birth**

_____   _____
Name of school   **Date of examination**

Professional evaluator: Licensed ophthalmologist or optometrist.

Based on my examination, _____ **(does/does not) appear to have**
                                         Name of student

a serious visual loss even after correction.

Exact measure of visual field and corrected visual acuity at distance and near in each eye:

Near: **Left**   **Right**

Distance: **Left**   **Right**

Visual field:

Type of impairment:

Severity of impairment:

Exact measurement could not be obtained. My best estimate is:

_____   _____   _____
Signature   **Position**   **Date**

ASSESSMENT DATA, ELIGIBILITY REPORT: VISUALLY HANDICAPPED

Part II

_____   _____   _____
Name of student   Chronological age   Date of birth

_____   _____
Name of school   Date of assessment

Professional evaluator: Certified educator of the visually handicapped or certified orientation and mobility instructor.

Procedures and results of functional and low vision assessment (must include performance of tasks in varied environments using both near and distant vision):

Implications for student's education:

_____   _____   _____
Signature   Position   Date

ASSESSMENT DATA ELIGIBILITY REPORT:
ORTHOPEDICALLY HANDICAPPED

_____   _____   _____
Name of student   **Chronological age**   **Date of birth**

_____   _____
Name of school   **Date of examination**

Professional evaluator: Licensed physician.

Based on my evaluation, _____ **(appears/does not appear) to**
                                          Name of student
have a severe orthopedic impairment that adversely affects educational performance.

Type of impairment:

Severity of impairment:

Functional implications of the handicapping condition for the educational process:

_____   _____
Signature of licensed physician   **Date**

ASSESSMENT DATA, ELIGIBILITY REPORT:
AUDITORIALLY HANDICAPPED (OTOLOGICAL REPORT)

Name of student   **Chronological age**   **Date of birth**

Name of school   **Date of examination**

Professional evaluator: Licensed otologist.

Based on my examination, _____ (does/does not) appear to have
                               Name of student

a serious hearing loss even after corrective medical treatment and/or use of amplification.

Type of impairment:

Severity of impairment:

Implications for student's education:

Signature   **Position**   **Date**

ASSESSMENT DATA, ELIGIBILITY REPORT:
AUDITORIALLY HANDICAPPED (AUDIOLOGICAL REPORT)

_____   _____   _____
Name of student   **Chronological age**   **Date of birth**

_____   _____
Name of school   **Date of assessment**

Professional evaluator: Licensed audiologist.

Results of audiological evaluation:

Implications of the hearing loss for the student's education in a variety of circumstances with or without recommended amplification. (Audiogram alone is not sufficient.) Specify (including speech reception threshold for students with residual hearing):

_____   _____   _____
Signature   **Position**   **Date**

ASSESSMENT DATA, ELIGIBILITY REPORT: DEAF-BLIND STUDENT

_____   _____   _____
Name of student   Chronological age   Date of birth

_____   _____
Name of school   Date of report

Auditorially Handicapped

Attached is a written report from an otologist that documents eligibility as an auditorially
handicapped student.

☐   ☐
Yes   **No**

_____   _____   _____
Name of evaluator   Position   Date of examination

Visually Handicapped

Attached is a written report from an ophthalmologist or optometrist that documents eligibility as a visually handicapped student.

☐   ☐
Yes   **No**

_____   _____   _____
Name of evaluator   Position   Date of examination

Functional Assessment

Attached are written reports (audiological and functional vision evaluations) that document
eligibility as auditorially and visually handicapped student.

☐   ☐
Yes   **No**

_____   _____   _____
Name of evaluator: Audiological   Position   Date of evaluation

_____   _____   _____
Name of evaluator: Functional vision   Position   Date of evaluation

Based on the reports cited, a hearing loss is   ☐ conclusively demonstrated.

☐ suspected but not demonstrated.

If a hearing loss is suspected, but not demonstrated, an attached speech/language evaluation indicates
that this student has no speech at an age when speech would normally be expected. ☐ Yes   ☐ No

_____   _____   _____
Name of evaluator: Certified speech therapist   Position   Date of evaluation

Person preparing this report:

_____   _____   _____
Signature   Position   Date

292

ASSESSMENT DATA, ELIGIBILITY REPORT: AUTISTIC STUDENT

_____   _____   _____
Name of student   **Chronological age**   **Date of birth**

_____   _____
Name of school   **Date of report**

Professional evaluators: Licensed physician or psychologist, certified speech therapist, and educational diagnostician or other evaluation specialist.

This student evidences the criteria for one of the following categories (as checked) of the pervasive developmental disorders (criteria from DSM III):

☐ **Infantile Autism**

    ☐ **Onset before 30 months of age.**

    ☐ **Pervasive lack of responsiveness to other people.**

    ☐ **Gross deficits in language development.**

    ☐ **If speech is present, peculiar speech patterns, such as immediate and delayed echolalia, metaphorical language, pronominal reversal.**

    ☐ **Bizarre responses to various aspects of the environment, e.g., resistance to change, peculiar interest in or attachments to animate or inanimate objects.**

    ☐ **Absence of delusions, hallucinations, loosening of associations, and incoherence as in schizophrenia.**

☐ **Infantile Autism, Residual State**

    ☐ **Once had an illness that met the criteria for infantile autism.**

    ☐ **The current clinical picture no longer meets the full criteria for infantile autism, but signs of the illness have persisted to the present, such as oddities of communication and social awkwardness.**

☐ **Childhood Onset Pervasive Developmental Disorder**

    ☐ **Gross and sustained impairment in social relationships, e.g., lack of appropriate affective responsivity, inappropriate clinging, asociality, lack of empathy.**

    ☐ **At least three of the following:**

        ☐ **Sudden excessive anxiety manifested by such symptoms as free-floating anxiety, catastrophic reactions to everyday occurrences, inability to be consoled when upset, unexplained panic attacks.**

        ☐ **Constricted or inappropriate affect, including lack of appropriate fear reactions, unexplained rage reactions, and extreme mood lability.**

        ☐ **Resistance to change in the environment (e.g., upset if dinner time is changed) or insistence on doing things in the same manner every time (e.g., putting on clothes always in same order).**

Childhood Onset Pervasive Developmental Disorder (continuation of listing on previous page)

☐ Oddities of motor movement, such as peculiar posturing, peculiar hand or finger movements, or walking on tiptoe.

☐ Abnormalities of speech, such as question like melody, monotonous voice.

☐ Hyper- or hyposensitivity to sensory stimuli, e.g., hyperacusis.

☐ Self-mutilation, e.g., biting or hitting self, head banging.

☐ Onset of the full syndrome after 30 months of age and before 12 years of age.

☐ Absence of delusions, hallucinations, incoherence, or marked loosening of associations.

☐ **Childhood Onset Pervasive Developmental Disorder, Residual State**

☐ Once had an illness that met the criteria for childhood onset pervasive developmental disorder.

☐ The current clinical picture no longer meets the full criteria for the disorder, but signs of the illness have persisted to the present, such as oddities of communication and social awkwardness.

☐ **Atypical pervasive developmental disorder**
This category should be used for children with distortions in the development of multiple basic psychological functions that are involved in the development of social skills and language and that cannot be classified as either infantile autism or childhood onset pervasive developmental disorder.

Comments:

Sources of data:

Specific recommendations for family counseling:

Specific recommendations for behavior management:

Multidisciplinary team:

Signature	Position	Concur	Dissent	Date
Licensed physician or psychologist				
Certified speech therapist				
Educational diagnostician or other evaluation specialist				

ASSESSMENT DATA, ELIGIBILITY REPORT: PREGNANT STUDENT

_____   _____   _____
Name of student   **Chronological age**   **Date of birth**

_____   _____
Name of school   **Date of examination**

Professional evaluator: Licensed physician.

_____ **is pregnant and is expected to deliver her baby**
Name of student
by approximately _____.
                     Date

Instructions: Complete the section below only _if student must be excused from compulsory school attendance._

Reason(s) this student should be excused from compulsory school attendance (including homebound classes). Specify temporary condition:

Treatment prescribed for this temporary condition:

Anticipated period of time for student's absence from school is from _____ **to**
_____.

_____   _____   _____
Signature   **Position**   **Date**

ASSESSMENT DATA, ELIGIBILITY REPORT: RELATED SERVICES

_____   _____   _____
Name of student   **Chronological age**   **Date of birth**

_____   _____
Name of school   **Date of assessment**

To be completed by professional evaluator: Registered, licensed, or certified related service provider.

Nature of Student's Problem

Specific Learning Competencies (include names of tests or procedure used to obtain data):

Degree of Severity of the Problem

Based on my assessment, _____ **(does/does not) need**
                            Name of student

_____ **to benefit from instruction.**
Name of related service

Related Services

Anticipated instructional benefits include

Recommended goals and objectives for the IEP include

Recommendations for service delivery (e.g., length and frequency of sessions; how and by whom should be delivered):

Signature of professional evaluator:

_____   _____   _____

Signature   **Position**   **Date**

ASSESSMENT DATA, ELIGIBILITY REPORT: OTHER HEALTH IMPAIRED

_____   _____   _____
Name of student   **Chronological age**   **Date of birth**

_____   _____
Name of school   **Date of examination**

Based on my examination, _____ (does/does not) appear to have
                                         Name of student

limited strength, vitality, or alertness, due to chronic or acute health problems which adversely affect
educational performance.

Type of impairment:

Severity of impairment:

**Implications for student's education (e.g., precautions regarding student's mobility, activity, cognitive
ability; need for rest periods and special equipment; effects of any medication; and need for medical
updates).**

_____   _____   _____
Signature   **Position**   **Date**

298

SPECIAL EDUCATION—NURSE'S WORKSHEET

Student	Grade	Screening assessment: Vision, hearing, classroom observation	Medical update	Health and developmental history	Quick neurological screening test	Physical assessment	School guidance meeting	IEP meeting	Annual/ triennial review	Comments

FORMS FOR
SPECIAL NURSING
PROCEDURES

The following forms provide permission to the school nurse to perform various special care procedures for children with disabilities or other problems that require hospital-related methods of management during school hours.

These forms are useful for the school nurse, occupational and physical therapists, and health aides and can be used under the following circumstances:

1. Children with tracheostomies that require suction and cleaning.
2. Children with abdominal ostomy bags that require daily cleaning and changing.
3. Children who require clean intermittent catheterization.
4. Children who require naso-gastric or other type of tube feeding.
5. Children who require pharyngeal suction due to excess secretions.
6. Children with fragile bones and joints who are in danger of spontaneous fracture and require positioning.
7. Children who require peritoneal dialysis.
8. Other unusual procedures that may be ordered by the student's physician.

The first form is initiated by the nurse by completing items 1 and 2. Items 3 through 9 are completed by the attending physician. The parent signature space and following information requested is to be added by the parent.

PHYSICIAN/PARENT REQUEST FOR ADMINISTRATION OF MEDICINE OR SPECIAL PROCEDURE BY SCHOOL PERSONNEL

Special health care procedures and medications may be prescribed for administration by school personnel as follows:

     1. When such treatment cannot otherwise be accomplished.

     2. On receipt of this completed form along with prescription and/or special equipment items.

Prescribed in-school medication/treatment may be administered by a nonhealth professional designate of the principal or school nurse.

1. Name of pupil _____ Birthdate _____

2. Address _____ School _____

3. Condition for which prescribed treatment is required:

4. Specific medication or procedure:

5. Dosage and method of administration:

6. Precautions, unfavorable reactions:

7. Disposition of pupil following administration or procedure, if applicable (i.e., rest, home, hospital, doctor's office, return to class):

8. Date of request _____ Date of termination _____

9. _____ / _____
    Physician's name (printed)   Signature

    _____ / _____
    Physician's address   Telephone number

(Parent)

We (I), the undersigned, the parents/guardians of _____
                                           Student's name

request the above medication or procedure be administered to our (my) child.

_____ / _____ Telephone _____ / _____
Name   Relationship   Home   Business

_____ / _____ Telephone _____ / _____
Name   Relationship   Home   Business

Filed in nurse's office on _____ by _____

Medication or Special Procedure Record

Student's name _____ Grade _____

1. Medication _____ Dosage _____ Time _____

2. Medication _____ Dosage _____ Time _____

Special procedure: _____
_____

After medication(s) or special procedure, record time(s) and initials in the appropriate week of month/day and date of week space. All medications must be on prescription of physician.

School name _____ School year _____

Week	Dates M/F	Time	August M	T	W	TH	F	Week	Dates M/F	Time	September M	T	W	TH	F	Week	Dates M/F	Time	October M	T	W	TH	F
1st								1st								1st							
2nd								2nd								2nd							
3rd								3rd								3rd							
4th								4th								4th							
5th								5th								5th							

Week	Dates M/F	Time	November M	T	W	TH	F	Week	Dates M/F	Time	December M	T	W	TH	F	Week	Dates M/F	Time	January M	T	W	TH	F
1st								1st								1st							
2nd								2nd								2nd							
3rd								3rd								3rd							
4th								4th								4th							
5th								5th								5th							

Week	Dates M/F	Time	February M	T	W	TH	F	Week	Dates M/F	Time	March M	T	W	TH	F	Week	Dates M/F	Time	April M	T	W	TH	F
1st								1st								1st							
2nd								2nd								2nd							
3rd								3rd								3rd							
4th								4th								4th							
5th								5th								5th							

Week	Dates M/F	Time	May M	T	W	TH	F	Week	Dates M/F	Time	June M	T	W	TH	F
1st								1st							
2nd															
3rd															
4th															
5th															

Disposition:

Prescription depleted _____

Medication or procedure discontinued _____

Medication returned to parents _____

Medication destroyed _____

Comments _____
_____
_____
_____
_____

PHYSICIAN'S AUTHORIZATION FOR HAVING SPECIALIZED PHYSICAL HEALTH CARE SERVICE PROCEDURES ADMINISTERED

Name of student _____ **Birthdate** _____

Address _____

1. Physical condition for which the standardized procedure is to be performed: _____
_____

2. Name of standardized procedure: _____

3. Precautions, possible untoward reactions, and interventions: _____
_____
_____

4. Time schedule and/or indication for the procedure: _____

5. The procedure is to be continued as above until: _____
Date

_____   _____
Physician's signature   Date

_____   _____
Address   Telephone

I hereby request that the treatment specified be performed to the above-named child.

_____   _____
Signature of parent/guardian   Date

SPECIALIZED PHYSICAL HEALTH CARE SERVICE—DAILY LOG OF TREATMENT ADMINISTERED

Name _____ **Birthdate** _____

School _____

Procedure _____

From _____, 19 ___ **To** _____, 19 ___

Physician _____ **Phone** _____

Date / /			Date / /			Date / /		
Time	Comment	Init.	Time	Comment	Init.	Time	Comment	Init.

Date / /			Date / /			Date / /		
Time	Comment	Init.	Time	Comment	Init.	Time	Comment	Init.

Date / /			Date / /			Date / /		
Time	Comment	Init.	Time	Comment	Init.	Time	Comment	Init.

Date / /			Date / /			Date / /		
Time	Comment	Init.	Time	Comment	Init.	Time	Comment	Init.

Date / /			Date / /			Date / /		
Time	Comment	Init.	Time	Comment	Init.	Time	Comment	Init.

Signatures	Title	Date

305

HEMATOCRIT AND URINALYSIS PERMISSION FORM

Student's name _____ D.O.B. _____

Room/teacher _____ School _____

Date _____

      The school district performs blood tests for anemia and a urine test for sugar and protein on students in selected grades in school. These tests are performed under the direction of the school nurse and the school physician and are free of charge.

      I do _____ do not _____ give permission for a blood test (hematocrit) for anemia and a urine test (urinalysis) for sugar and protein.

_____
Signature of parent or guardian

PERMISSION FOR EXTERNAL AUDITORY CANAL IRRIGATION

Dear Parent,

Your child _____ has been found to have a large amount of wax buildup in his ear canals. Since this may affect his or her ability to hear well, the wax should be removed. You may take your child to your family doctor or you may request that the school nurse carry out the procedure for removing the wax.

If you wish this procedure to be done by the school nurse please answer the following questions and sign below.

   1. Does your child have frequent earaches?

               _____ Yes   _____ No

   2. Have you noticed drainage from your child's ears?

               _____ Yes   _____ No

   3. Has your child ever had "tubes" placed in his ears by a doctor?

               _____ Yes   _____ No

   4. Has your child seen a doctor for ear problems during the last year?

               _____ Yes   _____ No

Although irrigation of the ears to remove wax is a safe and simple procedure, there is a possibility that your child could experience some slight irritation of the ear canals and/or some dizziness that lasts for a short while. For these reasons we ask that a parent be present during the procedure. The nurse will notify you when she schedules the procedure. If you have any questions, please call the school nurse.

_____ **Yes, I would like to have the school nurse irrigate my child's ears and agree to be present while it is being done. I understand that drops to soften the wax will be used prior to the irrigation.**

_____ **No, I do not want the nurse to irrigate my child's ear. I will take my child to our family doctor.**

_____
Parent's signature

_____
Date

PARENTAL NOTIFICATION OF TUBERCULOSIS TEST

Dear Parent:

The Health Department, in cooperation with local school officials, is conducting a tuberculin testing program of students in the _____ and _____ grades. The tuberculin test is simple and painless. It consists of placing a harmless test solution into the skin to show whether or not your child is infected with the germs that cause tuberculosis.

Your child may have the test only if you fill in and sign the Permission Form on the reverse side and have the child return it to the school without delay. It is *very important* to list the names of all people living in the home.

Experience in the past shows that most of the tests are negative, which is a welcome assurance that your child is not infected with tuberculosis germs. If you do not receive a report within three weeks after the test was made, you can assume the test was negative.

When the Permission Form has been signed, please have it returned to the classroom teacher. We appreciate your cooperation.

Sincerely yours,

TUBERCULOSIS TEST PERMISSION FORM

School _____

Child's name _____ Teacher _____

Mailing address _____

Birthdate _____ Telephone _____

Any previous TB skin tests? _____ Yes _____ No   If Yes, date _____ Results _____

Has any member of the household ever been a patient at the Chest Clinic? _____ Yes _____ No

If Yes, please list the name of this person _____

I give permission for the tuberculin test(s) and chest X ray, if necessary, for the protection of my child. I understand this is a free service.

_____
Signature of parent or guardian

Instructions: Please complete the following:

Doctor we usually go to _____

Doctor's address _____

People living in the home

Name	Birthdate
_____	_____
_____	_____
_____	_____
_____	_____
_____	_____
_____	_____

Parents: Leave this space blank.

Follow-up study	Result
_____	_____
_____	_____
_____	_____
_____	_____
_____	_____

(Please do not write below this line.)

(Please leave lines above blank.)

Heaf test

Date	Results

Mantoux test

Date	Measurement induration

HEALTH CARE MANAGEMENT FOR THE CHILD WITH SEIZURES

I. Remain calm

1. Lay the child down on his side so the tongue cannot fall back in the mouth. Place something soft under the head. Do *not* put anything in the mouth.

2. Do not try physically to stop the seizure.

3. Restrain the child just enough to prevent injury by falling or hitting the head. Do not hold the child down with force.

4. Stay with child throughout seizure.

5. Do not attempt to give anything by mouth during seizure.

6. It is commonplace for a child to hold his breath when having a seizure. If the child stops breathing for longer than 2 minutes, start mouth to mouth resuscitation. If the child does not start breathing, tell someone to call emergency ambulance, and resume mouth-to-mouth breathing until it arrives, or until the child starts breathing alone.

7. Write down how long the seizure lasted and describe it (eyes rolling to one side, jerking of arms and legs, vomiting, etc.).

8. If seizures become different, worse, or more frequent, consult a doctor.

9. Following the seizure, clean the child up if necessary.

10. If he is drowsy, allow him to sleep.

11. Offer nothing by mouth until he seems back to normal consciousness.

12. Explain to child, in words he can understand, what has happened to him and allow him to ask questions or talk about any feelings he might have.

II. Medication therapy: The immediate goal is to control seizures completely. Consider the following primary antiepileptic drugs currently in most common use.

Generic (trade name)	Indications	Average daily maintenance dose (mg/kg)		Most common side effects	Most common toxic signs and symptoms
		Adults	Children		
Phenobarbital (luminal)	Generalized tonic-clonic seizures; all forms of partial seizures	2–3	3–5	Sedation, parodoxical excitement, rash, irritability, and hyperactivity, especially in children	Drowsiness, ataxia, nystagmus, slurred speech
Phenytoin (Dilatin)	Generalized tonic-clonic seizures; all forms of partial seizures	3–5	4–7	Skin eruptions, hypergingival hyperplasia, coarsening of facial features, decreased blood folate level, hypocalcemia osteomalacia, lymphadenopathy hepatitis, systemic lupus erythematosus, fever	Nystagmus, ataxia, slurred speech, drowsiness, diplopia, blurred vision
Primidone	Generalized tonic-clonic seizures, all forms of partial seizures	10–25	10–25	Same as phenobarbital	Same as phenobarbital
Ethosuximide (Zarontin)	Petit mal seizures	20–40	20–30	Nausea, skin rash, blood dyscrasia, drowsiness, hiccups	Nausea, vomiting anorexia, lethargy, headache, hiccups
Carbamazepine	All forms of partial seizures; generalized tonic-clonic seizures	10–20	20–30	Nausea, vomiting, anorexia, blood dyscrasia	Vertigo, drowsiness, nystagmus, diplopia, unsteadiness
Valproic acid (Depakene)	Petit mal seizures, mixed seizures with petit mal	30–60	30–60	Nausea, vomiting, drowsiness, weight gain, transient alopecia, hypersalivation, diarrhea, thrombocytopenia, hepatic toxicity	Ataxia, sedation

III. Consider the needs of the whole patient: the goal, along with better seizure control should be improved family and social relationships

HYPERTENSION SCREENING

Hypertension is a significant public health problem in the United States. Prevalence rates vary by age, race, nutrition, environmental stresses, and certain physical health problems. The incidence of hypertension in school-age children is very low; therefore, the value of screening large numbers of children is questioned by some authorities. However, for those school districts that conduct screening programs, the following guidelines will be helpful.

Procedures and Techniques

- Seat the child facing the screener with the forearm suitably bared and resting on a table.
- Apply the appropriate cuff size, leaving a space of about 1 cm between the bottom of the cuff and the elbow.
- Locate the brachial artery pulse by palpation and place the diaphragm of the stethoscope over the artery. Rapidly inflate the cuff and deflate gradually until the first clear tapping sound is heard. Record this point as the systolic pressure. Continue to deflate the cuff while the sound becomes clearer, louder, and crisper, then suddenly changes to a low-pitched muffled one, then disappears. Record the diastolic pressure at the point the sound suddenly changes to a muffled tone (ex: 100/80).

Cuff size must be individualized for each child. The bladder of the cuff should be two-thirds of the distance from the elbow to the axilla (armpit). Obese children are usually taller than average and need a larger and longer cuff.

For normal blood pressure ranges, see graphs.

Standard for Referral

If the systolic and/or diastolic pressure is frequently at the 90th percentile for age or at the 95th percentile on one or more occasion, the student should be referred. Unusually high or low readings should be rechecked after student has had a chance to rest in the school clinic.

PERCENTILES OF BLOOD PRESSURE MEASUREMENT

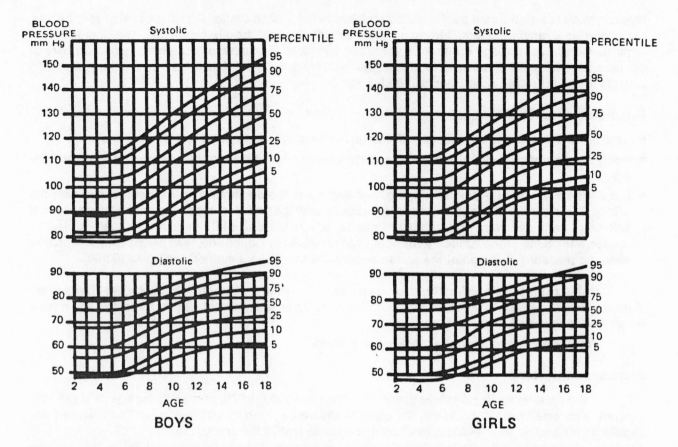

The numbers to the right of each square are percentiles. Average is 50 percent and anything between 5th and 95th percentile is considered normal (very low—under 5—or very high—over 95—is not normal). Readings of 90 to 95 percent should be followed carefully and referred to a physician if scores remain high. Low readings have no significance unless accompanied by symptoms such as fainting.

Reproduced by permission of *Pediatrics,* Vol. 59, p. 5. Copyright © 1977 by *Pediatrics.*

FORMS FOR
SUPPLIES

REQUISITION FOR SCHOOL HEALTH SERVICES FORMS

The Requisition for School Health Services Forms would of course have to be adapted for your particular school system. It is given here only as an example.

Health service forms should be used by the nurse to maintain an appropriate number of each of the forms applicable to grade-level population and nurse role function in each building.

CLINIC INVENTORY

A new Clinic Inventory should be completed during the opening week of school. Compare the new school year inventory with last year's copy of the inventory to note any significant differences in totals.

REQUISITION FOR SCHOOL HEALTH SERVICES FORMS

_____ H-2   Health History (English/Spanish)

_____ H-4   Head Injury—Parent Letter (English/Spanish) (50 sheets per pad)

_____ H-5   Pediculosis Control—Parent Letter (English/Spanish) (50 sheets per pad)

_____ H-6   Medical Report from School (English/Spanish) (50 sheets per pad)

_____ H-7   Health Care Monitoring and Teaching Record for Pregnant Students

_____ H-8   Immunization Requirements—Parent Letter (Spanish)

_____ H-9   Impedance Report Log

_____ H-10   Health Status and Care Plan (Keypunch)

_____ H-11   Substitute Nurse—Verification of Assignment

_____ H-16   Medical Referral/Follow-up Form

_____ H-17   Medical Report (English/Spanish)

_____ H-18   Health History Worksheet

_____ H-19   SNP Pathology File

_____ H-20   Student Health Assessment Activities (Keypunch)

_____ H-21   Incident Report

_____ H-22   Appointment Slip (Spanish) (20 to a pad)

_____ H-23   Send to Clinic (100 sheets per pad)

_____ H-24   Appointment Slips (English) (100 sheets per pad)

_____ H-25   Pupil's Referral Slip (for Elementary Schools)

_____ H-26   HMP for Student with Seizures

_____ H-27   Record of Clinic Visits (for Secondary Schools)

_____ H-29   Health Summary Card

_____ H-37   Accident Report Form (Keypunch)

_____ H-38   Request for School Health Services

_____ H-40   Application for Lions Club Services

_____ H-43   Schedule of Nurses Work (6 weeks)

_____ H-44   Clinic Inventory

_____ H-45   Nurse's Daily Schedule of Activities

_____ H-47   Pure-Tone Hearing Test

_____ H-48   Monthly Hearing Report

_____ H-54   Health Management Plan

_____ H-55   Health Record (Cumulative)

_____ H-56   Medical Evaluation

_____ H-56C&Y Children and Youth

_____ H-56E Vision Evaluation for Developmentally Delayed Students

_____ H-56H Conners' Report

_____ H-57   Parent Permission to Examine

_____ H-57A Records Release Authorization (Requesting information about students)

_____ H-57B Records Release Authorization (Requesting information about employees)

_____ H-57C Records Release Authorization (for DISD to release information)

_____ H-58   Nurse's Report of Communicable Disease

_____ H-60   Referral Audiogram (50 per pad)

_____ H-61   Principal's Notice of Hearing Technician's Schedule

_____ H-62   Results from Electoacoustic Impedance Measurement

_____ H-63   Student's Request for Excused Health Care Absence (100 sheets per pad)

Date _____

Box # _____

Nurse _____

School _____

MEDICAL SUPPLY ORDER FORM (ANNUAL)

School _____ Date _____

The supplies listed below are obtained from Central Office Health Services. Please estimate the quantities you will obtain in August prior to the beginning of school.

Item	Description	Quantity Estimate
Ace bandage	2"	_____
Ace bandage	3"	_____
Bandaids	box	_____
Bandage rolls	3"	_____
Cotton balls	bag	_____
Forceps, splinter	4½"	_____
Forceps, thumb	4½"	_____
Plastic bags and ties	17½" x 8½"	_____
Q-tips	100 per pkg.	_____
Scissors		_____
Slings, arm		_____
Splints (basswood)		_____
Steri-pad	4" x 4"	_____
Telfa pad	3" x 4"	_____
Thermometers		_____
Therapeutic preparations		
Bacitracin	1 oz.	_____
Calamine lotion	8 oz.	_____
Lubriderm	4 oz.	_____
Urinalysis		
Uristix		_____
Urine cups		_____
Microlance (hematocrits)		_____
Glass pipettes		_____
Seal-ease		_____
Linen		
Bed sheet	72" x 108"	_____
Bedspread		_____
Blanket		_____
Pillow		_____
Pillowcase	42" x 36"	_____

Please order no more than two each of the medical supplies listed below. Orders of $10.00 or more will be delivered to the schools.

Item	Description	Unit	No. wanted
Alcohol	Rubbing	Bottle	_____
Ammonia	Spirits	Bottle	_____
Cotton	Absorbent	Box	_____
Eugenol	1 oz.	Bottle	_____
Foille	1 oz.	Bottle	_____
Merthiolate	Stainless	Pint bottle	_____
Ointment	Desenex 9 oz.	Tube	_____
Powder	Desenex 1½ oz.	Can	_____
Soap	Septisol	Gallon	_____
Tape	Adhesive	6 rolls to box	_____
Tongue depressors	500 (Junior)	Box	_____
Tongue depressors	500 (Regular)	Box	_____
Vaseline	White	Jar	_____

CLINIC INVENTORY

School _____ **Date** _____

	Opening of school (date)	Close of school (date)
Health supplies		
Alcohol, rubbing compound	_____	_____
Ammonia, spirits of aromatic	_____	_____
Antiseptic, Wescodyne, 1-gal.	_____	_____
Applicator, tooth pick round	_____	_____
Bandaid, ¾" x 3"	_____	_____
Bandage, gauze 1" x 10 yd	_____	_____
Bandage, gauze 2" x 10 yd	_____	_____
Bandage, triangular 37" x 37" x 52"	_____	_____
Basin, emesis porcelain	_____	_____
Basin, wash porcelain	_____	_____
Betadine, antiseptic solution	_____	_____
Binders, 8½" x 5½" 3-ring	_____	_____
Blanket, cotton 72" x 84" 1½ lb.	_____	_____
Box, file activity #94	_____	_____
Cap, ice	_____	_____
Case, pillow muslin 42" x 36"	_____	_____
Chart, letters, HOTV	_____	_____
Chart, Snellen Plastic #LD-25 direct	_____	_____
Chart, Snellen plastic mirror #L1-25	_____	_____
Chart, Snellen plastic #E-25	_____	_____
Chart, Snellen #V-3 line of letters	_____	_____
Chart, Snellen mir. for line of letters	_____	_____
Chart, vision testing 9" x 14" HOTV	_____	_____
Balls, cotton medium 2,000 to pkg	_____	_____
Covers, Snellen #V-5	_____	_____
Cup. drink strgt. edge cone type 4 oz.	_____	_____
Depressor, tongue senior	_____	_____
Fillers, white three-hole 8½" x 5½"	_____	_____
Pad, gauze surgical 2" x 2"	_____	_____
Gauze, surgical 1 yd x 5 yds	_____	_____
Guide, card A-Z plain 5th cut 6" x 4"	_____	_____
Kit, first aid	_____	_____
Kwell, pediculosis 1-gal	_____	_____
Lens, plus	_____	_____
Mirror, dental #4	_____	_____
Oil of cloves, 4 oz	_____	_____
Pad, heating electric	_____	_____
Paper, examination table, white	_____	_____
RID	_____	_____
Sheet, muslin 54" x 99"	_____	_____
Signals, Nu-Vise, assorted	_____	_____
Soap, hand 3 oz.	_____	_____
Splint, wood 3½" x 18"	_____	_____
Stethoscope, single prong medium	_____	_____
Tape, adhesive ½" x 10 yds	_____	_____
Tape, adhesive 1" x 10 yds	_____	_____
Thermometer #BO oral	_____	_____
Tip, "Q" nonsterile (100 to pkg)	_____	_____
Tray, instrument porcelain	_____	_____
Tweezers, diagonal tip	_____	_____
Vaseline, plain ⅜ oz	_____	_____
Scissors, sharp point 5"	_____	_____
Other	_____	_____

	Opening of school (date)	Close of school (date)
Furniture and equipment		
Black light for ringworm screening	_____	_____
Chairs	_____	_____
Cot	_____	_____
Couch	_____	_____
Covered waste receptacles	_____	_____
Desk (describe kind)	_____	_____
Enamel-top table	_____	_____
Filing cabinet	_____	_____
Goose-neck lamp	_____	_____
Mattress	_____	_____
Measuring stand	_____	_____
Mirror	_____	_____
Mobile record and supply cabinet	_____	_____
Pillow	_____	_____
Policies and procedures manual	_____	_____
Pseudo-isochromatic color vision plates	_____	_____
Scales, bathroom	_____	_____
Scales, platform	_____	_____
Sphygmomanometers	_____	_____
Stool	_____	_____
Stretcher	_____	_____
Three-panel screen	_____	_____
Vision test chart, lighted	_____	_____
Other	_____	_____
_____	_____	_____
_____	_____	_____
_____	_____	_____

_____   _____
Nurse's signature   Nurse's signature

SUPPLY REQUEST FORM

School _____ Date requested _____

Nurse _____ Date to be picked up _____ / _____

| | A.M. | P.M. |

Item _____ **No. requested** _____ **No. issued**

_____

_____

_____

_____

_____

_____

_____

_____

_____

_____

_____

_____

_____

_____

_____

_____

_____

_____

_____

_____

_____

_____

_____

_____

_____

_____

_____

_____

FORMS FOR TEACHER-NURSE CONSULTATIONS

PLEASE SEND TO CLINIC FORM

The Please Send to Clinic form is completed by the nurse or nurse designate to advise the teacher of a student's nurse-initiated visit to the clinic.

REFERRALS TO THE SCHOOL NURSE

The Referrals to the School Nurse may be used by the school nurse to record referrals from an individual teacher or by the teacher to record all of his or her referrals to the health clinic.

STUDENT'S REQUEST FOR EXCUSED HEALTH CARE ABSENCE

The Student's Request for Excused Health Care Absence may be used by primary health care providers when students make appointments during school time. The school nurse may give a form to the student when she gives a referral, if appropriate.

PUPIL'S REFERRAL SLIP

The following Pupil's Referral Slip is filled out by the elementary teacher and is sent with the student to the principal or nurse in case of an accident or suspected illness. One copy should be filed in the clinic; another may be used to send information concerning the student back to the teacher or to the principal by the nurse.

PLEASE SEND TO CLINIC

_____

Please send _____

_____

to the clinic at (once) (close of class) (teacher's convenience).

Date _____   _____

GUIDE FOR TEACHER'S REFERRAL TO NURSE

It is recommended that the following observations be referred to the nurse:

Eyes
a. Sties or crusted eyelids
b. Inflammed eyelids
c. Crossed eyes
d. Repeated headaches
e. Squinting, frowning, or scowling
f. Protruding eyes
g. Watery eyes
h. Rubbing of eyes
i. Twitching of the lids
j. Excessive blinking
k. Holding head to one side
l. Complaints of blurry vision

Teeth and mouth
a. State of uncleanliness
b. Gross caries
c. Irregular teeth
d. Stained teeth
e. Gum boils
f. Offensive breath
g. Mouth habits such as thumb sucking
h. Complaints of toothache
i. Swollen jaw

Heart
a. Excessive breathlessness
b. Tires easily
c. Any history of "growing pains"
d. Bluish lips or fingernails
e. Excessive pallor

Growth
a. Failure to gain regularly over 6-month period
b. Unexplained loss in weight
c. Unexplained rapid gain in weight

Ears
a. Discharge from ears
b. Earache
c. Failure to hear questions
d. Picking at the ears
e. Turning head to hear
f. Talking in a monotone
g. Inattention
h. Anxious expression
i. Excessive noisiness of child
j. Ringing in ears
k. Dizziness

Glands
a. Enlarged glands at side of neck
b. Enlarged thyroid

General appearance and condition
a. Underweight, very thin
b. Overweight, very obese
c. Does not appear well
d. Tires easily
e. Chronic fatigue
f. Nausea or vomiting
g. Faintness or dizziness
h. Chronic menstrual discomfort

Posture and musculature
a. Alignment of shoulders
b. Peculiarity of gait
c. Obvious deformities of any type
d. Alignment of spine on "standing tall"
e. Muscular development
f. Coordination
g. Muscle tone
h. Use of feet in standing and walking

Nose and throat
a. Persistent mouth breathing
b. Frequent sore throats
c. Recurrent colds
d. Chronic nasal discharge
e. Frequent nose bleeding
f. Nasal speech
g. Frequent tonsilitis
h. Chronic coughing

Any chronic illness (known or suspected diagnosis)
a. Diabetes
b. Epilepsy
c. Rheumatic fever
d. Cystic fibrosis
e. Orthopedic condition
f. Severe hearing loss
g. Unremedial visual loss or handicap
h. Other special conditions

Other
a. Students who lack medical care due to financial stress or religious views
b. Known or suspected social, family, financial situations affecting the health of the student
c. Prolonged absenteeism due to illness
d. Homebound students
e. Suspected or known pregnancies
f. Children subjected to physical abuse
g. Children receiving medications for a prolonged time and for chronic conditions
h. Students new to school district

Skin and scalp
a. Unusual pallor of face
b. Eruptions or rashes
c. Habitual scratching of scalp or skin
d. Nits on the hair
e. State of uncleanliness
f. Excessive redness of face

Behavior
a. Overstudious, docile, withdrawing
b. Bullying, overaggressiveness, and domineering
c. Unhappy and depressed
d. Overexcitable, uncontrollable emotions
e. Stuttering or other forms of speech difficulty
f. Poor accomplishment in comparison with ability
g. Lying (imaginative or defensive)
h. Lack of appreciation of property rights
i. Abnormal sex behavior
j. Antagonistic, negativistic, continual quarreling
k. Excessive use of toilet
l. Enuresis

TEACHER NOTIFICATION OF STUDENT'S HEALTH STATUS

_____, who is enrolled in your class, has a health problem:

Name

_____

_____

_____

_____

Grade _____ **First Semester** _Instructions: Please initial below and pass to the next teacher._

Teacher	Class	Initial
_____	_____	_____
_____	_____	_____
_____	_____	_____
_____	_____	_____
_____	_____	_____
_____	_____	_____

Grade _____ **Second Semester** _Instructions: Please initial below and pass to the next teacher._

Teacher	Class	Initial
_____	_____	_____
_____	_____	_____
_____	_____	_____
_____	_____	_____
_____	_____	_____
_____	_____	_____

If you have questions regarding this, please ask me for further information. When all have signed, return to my mailbox.

_____

School nurse

REFERRALS TO THE SCHOOL NURSE

School _____ Teacher _____ Room _____

Date	Child's name	Reason for referral	Nurse's findings
____	_____	_____	_____
____	_____	_____	_____
____	_____	_____	_____
____	_____	_____	_____
____	_____	_____	_____
____	_____	_____	_____
____	_____	_____	_____
____	_____	_____	_____
____	_____	_____	_____
____	_____	_____	_____
____	_____	_____	_____
____	_____	_____	_____
____	_____	_____	_____
____	_____	_____	_____
____	_____	_____	_____
____	_____	_____	_____
____	_____	_____	_____
____	_____	_____	_____
____	_____	_____	_____
____	_____	_____	_____
____	_____	_____	_____
____	_____	_____	_____
____	_____	_____	_____
____	_____	_____	_____
____	_____	_____	_____
____	_____	_____	_____
____	_____	_____	_____
____	_____	_____	_____
____	_____	_____	_____
____	_____	_____	_____

STUDENT'S REQUEST FOR EXCUSED HEALTH CARE ABSENCE

_____   _____   _____
          Student name   **School address**   **Gr. section**

In response to ☐ **School referral by nurse/other**

                  ☐ **Acute care for illness/injury**

                  ☐ **Scheduled care initiated by provider/parent/student**

The above-named student was/will be **absent for** dental/medical **care as shown below:**

Date: ___/___/___   **Time:** _____/_____
              mo day yr   from   to

A follow-up appointment is/is not **scheduled (date where applicable** ___/___/___ **time** _____ **)**
                                                   mo day yr

Request for excused absence is made necessary because of

        ☐ **Urgency of health care need**

        ☐ **Appropriate appointment could not be arranged outside of school hours**

_____   _____
Parent signature   **Dentist/physician signature**

_____   _____
Date   **Telephone**   **Date**

PUPIL'S REFERRAL SLIP

Name _____ Grade _____ Time left room _____

Pupil's phone number _____ Date _____ Teacher _____

Shows the sign(s) or symptom(s) checked below:

☐ Asthma/wheezing ☐ Fever ☐ Nosebleed ☐ Stomachache

☐ Coughing/sneezing ☐ Headache ☐ Rash/skin condition ☐ Toothache

☐ Earache ☐ Nausea/vomiting ☐ Sore throat ☐ Wound

Other _____

Nurse's findings and recommendations _____

☐ Return to class ☐ Rest in clinic ☐ Permit to go home

Time left clinic _____ _____

Nurse

REFERRAL OF PUPIL TO NURSE BY TEACHER

Name _____ Grade _____ Date _____ Time _____

Instructions: Check or write reason for referral to nurse.

1. **Readmission after illness** _____
2. **Cold** _____
3. **Sore throat** _____
4. **Cough** _____
5. **Rash** _____
6. **Injury** _____
7. **Teeth** _____

8. **Eyes** _____
9. **Ears** _____
10. **Headache** _____
11. **Stomach** _____
12. **Hair** _____
13. **Other** _____

Teacher _____

Nurse's disposition of case:

Temperature _____
Taken home _____
Sent home _____

Returned to class _____
Taken to doctor _____

------detach--- detach--- detach------

Report to Teacher From Nurse

Name _____ Grade _____ Date _____ Time _____

1. Temperature _____
2. Taken home _____
3. Return to classroom _____

4. Rest on cot _____
5. Sent home _____
6. Return to nurse at _____

Remarks _____

Nurse _____

FORMS FOR VISION

Vision evaluation is required by most states for *all* special education students. For some with severe disabilities, the school nurse can only estimate the degree of visual impairment and, in many cases, must refer the child to an eye specialist. To evaluate this type child, school nurses receive special didactic and hands-on supervised experience. In some districts, this task is delegated to the school nurse practitioner.

Many students in this category do not have a refractive error that requires glasses; instead, the child lacks visual perception due to brain damage. Therefore, it is best to refer these children to a physician(s) who can do a thorough evaluation.

VISION EVALUATION FOR DEVELOPMENTALLY DELAYED STUDENTS

To complete the Vision Evaluation for Developmentally Delayed Students and prior to referral to a physician, some specialized inservice training plus supervised hands-on experience is necessary. It is recommended that this be done by a professional school nurse.

REPORT OF EYE INJURY

Many states have laws that require school districts to report eye injuries. Accumulated evidence of how and where the injuries occur leads to more effective safety measures.

Usually the school nurse is responsible for filling out the following Report of Eye Injury. In some districts, however, any authorized official may do so. For legal reasons, it is best to designate a certificated school person with some health-related training or background.

APPLICATION FOR LIONS CLUB SERVICES

Some civic organizations, such as the Lions Club, have, as a community service, some funding available for students who cannot obtain vision exams and/or eyeglasses. The application and explanatory letter might be distributed to parents.

PARENTAL NOTIFICATION OF RESULTS OF VISION/HEARING SCREENING EXAMINATION

The Parental Notification of Results of Vision/Hearing Screening Examination can be used for either the vision or hearing screening program. The next two forms are used for vision only. All three samples should be used to report only abnormal results of the problems mentioned on the forms. If the student has an eye or ear abnormality, such as pink eye or otitis media, the referral form in Section Sixteen may be used.

The Snellen 10- or 20-foot test chart is recommended by most experts as the preferred visual acuity test. One reason is that the examiner can see the eyes during the test to observe directly any deviation of either or both eyes.

ANNUAL VISION SCREENING SURVEY

In many states, vision testing is legally required for school attendance, and each district must submit an annual report, usually to the state health department.

Some states require only visual acuity testing; others require eye screening procedures for latent hyperopia, muscle imbalance, color vision, and depth perception.

Each school campus can use the following Annual Vision Screening Survey. When the forms are all collected and added together, they represent the district total. For maximum effectiveness, the district totals should be compared to national norms. Also, any significant annual deviation from year to year or from campus to campus should be scrutinized for possible error in screening.

VISION EVALUATION FOR DEVELOPMENTALLY DELAYED STUDENTS

Instructions: Please return in mail to director of School Health Services if information is confidential. Otherwise, return through channel received.

Name of pupil _____
              Last   **First**   **Middle**

Birthdate _____ Date of testing _____

School _____
                  Home school (or school attended, if different)

Home phone _____ Home address _____

Office phone _____

Significant history relative to vision (circle findings):

Note presence of any of the following symptoms:

Unequal pupils	Red eyes	Crusting of lids
Shuts or covers one eye frequently	Watery eyes or discharges	Photophobia
Tilts head to one side	Excessive eye rubbing	Styes or swollen lids
Blinks continually	Nystagmus	Other (explain)
Holds work close	Ptosis	No abnormalities noted

Estimate of Vision

Fixation on light _____

    Right eye (left eye covered) _____

    Left eye (right eye covered) _____

Picks up raisin (or similar size object) _____

Estimate of Alignment

Symmetrical corneal light reflex (Hirschberg) _____

Eye Disease

Gross lens/corneal opacities _____

    Red reflex _____

    Fundoscopic _____

       This examination (does, does not) suggest evidence of eye disease or vision impairment.

       This student (is, is not) being referred to a physician.

Physician's Findings

  I. Vision _____

 II. Alignment _____

III. Eye disease _____

    Diagnosis _____

    Recommendations _____

_____

_____   _____   _____
         Date   **Office telephone**   **Physician's signature**

*Reliable visual acuity not obtainable by tumbling E, HOTV, or other screening method.

REPORT OF EYE INJURY

_____
District name

_____
School name

Planned use of data: Establish preventive standards for schools, and development of safety education curriculum.
Instructions: Please prepare within five days of the eye injury and forward to _____
Address
if further clarification is needed.

1. **Name of injured** _____
   ( ) **Pupil**
   ( ) **Teacher**
   ( ) **Other** _____

2. **Sex** _____ **Age** _____ **Grade or position** _____

3. **Date of accident** _____ **Time of day** _____

4. **Time lost due to accident** _____

5. **Location of accident: School** _____ **Facility** _____

6. **Course being taught** _____

7. **Activity in class** _____

8. **Was activity supervised?** _____ **Yes** _____ **No**

9. **Name of supervisor or teacher** _____

10. **Nature and extent of injury** _____

    _____

11. **Cause of accident** _____

12. **Were protective eye devices worn?** _____ **Yes** _____ **No**

Typed Name of Authorized School Official	Telephone	Date

Signature of authorized school official

APPLICATION FOR LIONS CLUB SERVICES

To be completed by the nurse and signed by the parent as indicated. An explanation to the parent concerning the information required on the form is generally necessary to ensure correct information.

Eligibility for routine referral to the Lions Club Clinic is to be based on an identified

Vision loss of 20/50 or greater in both eyes or a two-line minimum difference between the visual acuity of each.

Strabismus, cataracts, corneal disease, old injury, or other significant medical history.

Documented financial hardship without resources for third-party pay.

When the form is complete, the school nurse should look at combined income, number of children, social history (outstanding debts, rent, utilities, medical bills, etc.), parent signature, and AFDC, to better determine need for assistance.

In the absence of financial hardship but with other factors that interfere with the likelihood of a student receiving appropriate visual examination, and/or correction, referral should be made to the area nurse for consideration of special approval for Lions Club assistance.

All applications should be sent to the area nurse for review and/or suggestions. Area nurses will send *complete* and *appropriate* referrals to Central Health Service.

APPLICATION FOR ASSISTANCE IN SECURING EYEGLASSES

I request help in securing vision examination and/or glasses for my child.

_____
Name of child

_____ _____ _____
School   Grade   Age

Visual examination done on _____ by _____ at _____
                                    Date   Examining doctor   Health facility

Assistance requested:

_____ Visual examination only   _____ Glasses only

_____ Visual examination and glasses

_____ Other. Specify _____

Social History:

Father _____ Occupation _____ Income _____

Soc. sec. no. _____

Mother _____ Occupation _____ Income _____

Soc. sec. no. _____

Number of children in family _____ Ages _____

Earnings of children employed _____

Other income _____

Aid to Families with
  Dependent Children (AFDC)   ☐ Yes   ☐ No

Social Security Insurance (SSI)   ☐ Yes   ☐ No

Medicaid   ☐ Yes   ☐ No

Other insurance   ☐ Yes   ☐ No

Other information or reasons why help is needed _____

_____

_____

I can contribute to the cost of my child's examination and/or glasses: ☐ Yes   ☐ No

$_____ now ☐   or monthly installments of $_____ per month.

_____   _____
School nurse   Parent signature

                                           _____
                                              Address

                                           _____
                                              Phone

334

PARENTAL NOTIFICATION OF RESULTS OF VISION/HEARING SCREENING EXAMINATION

To the parents of _____ Date of birth _____
                                    Student's name

A recent vision/hearing screening examination showed that your child should be checked more
            (circle one)
thoroughly by a vision/hearing specialist. If you have any questions or need any help, feel free to consult
            (circle one)
with the school nurse. See reverse side for results of screening.

_____   _____
School nurse   School

_____   _____
Date   Telephone no.

Specialist's Report to School Nurse

In addition to your medical diagnosis, will you please detail for the classroom teacher any modifications of the regular school program that may be helpful in this student's education (e.g., special seating, repetition of instruction, special materials). Student may return this form to the school nurse, or it may be mailed to

_____
School   Dept.   Address

_____

_____

_____

_____

_____

_____   _____
Physician's printed name   Physician's signature

_____   _____
Office phone   Date

PARENTAL NOTIFICATION OF RESULTS OF VISION/HEARING SCREENING EXAMINATION
Page 2

_____
Student's name

Note to Vision/Hearing Specialist
(Circle one.)

The above-named child has been referred because of

☐ A primary defect discovered during routine screening exams

☐ A learning problem that may be related to a visual or auditory problem

☐ Other_____

_____

Results of Vision Screening Exam:

Visual acuity

Without glasses R _____ L _____

With glasses   R _____ L _____

Test method used

Snellen 10' _____ 20' _____

Titmus _____

Other _____

Latent hyperopia (+2.5 lens)

☐ Passed   ☐ Failed   ☐ Not tested

Muscle imbalance (cover test)

☐ Passed   ☐ Failed   ☐ Not tested

Other_____

_____

Results of Hearing Screening Exam

Impedance bridge screening

☐ abnormal   ☐ Normal   ☐ Not performed

Audiogram (attached)

R   ☐ Passed   ☐ Failed   ☐ Not performed

L   ☐ Passed   ☐ Failed   ☐ Not performed

Other _____

_____

REPORT OF EYE EXAMINATION

Name of child _____ School _____ Date _____

Dear Parent:

As a result of a recent vision screening program at school we believe that your child should have a complete eye examination. We urge you to give this your prompt attention. Please take this form to your eye examiner and ask him to complete it and return it to the school. If you desire additional information, our school nurse will be happy to help you.

_____   _____
                Nurse   **Principal**

Note to the examiner:

We have directed the parents' attention to the need for complete examination because of:

Performance on Snellen test   Right 20/_____   Left 20/_____

Signs and symptoms _____

_____

_____

_____

The school will appreciate a report from you and any recommendations you desire to make. This information will be of help in planning the educational program for this child.

_____
            Student's name

Report of Examiner to the School

Visual acuity		**Glasses**

Without lenses   **With lenses**   ☐ **Not prescribed**

Right 20/_____ Left 20/_____   Right 20/_____ Left 20/_____   ☐ **Prescribed**

Both 20/_____   Both 20/_____   ☐ **To be worn all the time.**

☐ **To be worn for close work only**

☐ **Safety lenses**

Preferential seating recommended _____

Special materials that would be helpful _____

Other recommendations or suggestions _____

Date patient should return for further examination _____

_____   _____   _____
         Signature   **Address**   **Date**

VISION SCREENING AND/OR EYE EXAMINATION

Attention Parent: Please present this certificate when enrolling your child in school for the first time. Regulations _____ **requires that every child have an eye examination or approved vision screening test prior to, or within 90 days after, entry into** _____ **school.**

State

School _____ **City** _____ **County** _____

Child's name _____ **Birthdate** _____ **Age** _____ **Sex** _____

Parent's name _____ **Telephone number** _____

Address _____ **Zip code** _____

Vision Screener Report

Instructions: Visual acuity screening is only a check of the sharpness of a child's vision and should not be interpreted as a substitute for a complete vision examination. A child who fails this screening should be referred to an eye specialist for a complete visual examination.

Visual acuity
First test

Screened with glasses? Yes ☐
No ☐

Screening results
Passed ☐
Failed ☐

☐ Snellen Chart
☐ Other: _____   _____
(Instrument)

> Right eye 20/_____
> Left eye   20/_____

Second test

☐ Snellen Chart
☐ Other: _____   _____
(Instrument)

Passed ☐
Failed, referred ☐

> Right eye 20/_____
> Left eye   20/_____

Observable signs _____

Other tests(s) _____

_____
Reason for referral to eye specialist

_____ _____ _____
Date   Vision screener   Organization responsible for screening

Eye Specialist Report

Visual acuity	Without correction	With correction
Right eye	20/_____	20/_____
Left eye	20/_____	20/_____

Problem(s) noted: _____

Please check if appropriate:

☐ **Recommendations**
   ☐ **Medical evaluation**
   ☐ **Glasses**
   ☐ **Contact lenses**
   ☐ **Other** _____
☐ **Reexamination advised**
   ☐ **Six months**
   ☐ **Twelve months**
   ☐ **Other** _____

Present date _____

Date of last examination _____

☐ **Corrective lens prescribed**
   ☐ **Constant wear**
   ☐ **Near vision only**
   ☐ **Far vision only**
   ☐ **May be removed for physical education**

Please print or stamp

Doctor's name _____

Address _____

City _____

_____
Doctor's signature

ANNUAL VISION SCREENING SURVEY

Instructions: Please submit after referrals are completed, but prior to summer vacation.

School _____ District _____ Nurse _____

Address _____ City _____ County _____ Average enrollment _____

Grade levels represented _____ Did volunteers help screen? _____ Were machines used? ☐ Yes ☐ No

Grade	1 Number screened	Number of "failures" on each test after rescreening					7 Total referred	8 Received glasses or treatment	9 Saw doctor; treatment not needed	10 Referrals not yet completed	11 Color deficiency		12 Referrals completed from last year*
		2 Visual acuity	3 Farsighted	Binocular vision		6 Depth perception					Screened	Failed	
				4 Far	5 Near (strabismus)								
Pre-K													
Sp Ed													
K													
1													
2													
3													
4													
5													
6													
7													
8													
9													
10													
11													
12													
Total													

Reason for Incomplete Referrals This Year

Summer appointment [Number]

Parents refused to seek exam [Number]

Won't wear [Number]

Moved [Number]

Known eye problem _____ [Number]

Other _____ [Number]

*This column should reflect number of students listed as incomplete referrals last year who were examined prior to September 1 of this school year.

VISION SCREENING REPORT FOR SCHOOL YEAR 19__-19__

Health screening facility _____ City _____ County _____

Grades	A Total number screened	B Screened with glasses*	C Number failed	D Failed, not referred	Examined by eye specialist		G Referred, no follow-up
					E No problem/ no treatment	F Treatment or observation	
Preschool							
Special Educ.							
K							
1							
2							
3							
4							
5							
6							
7							
8							
9							
10							
11							
12							

C = D + E + F + G

Totals	A	B	C	D	E	F	G

Total examined by eye specialist
(E + F)

*This number is included in the total number screened and is, therefore, a smaller number.

To be submitted by June 30, 19____

To: Vision, Hearing, and Speech Services
Department of Health

_____
Chief administrator's signature

_____
Chief administrator's title

340

Instructions

Reporting period: September through August of the year prior to the reporting date.

Reporting date: June 30 following the reporting period.

Explanation of Columns

Grades: This column is self-explanatory. For preschools and other organizations screening preschool-aged children, simply enter totals on the line for preschool and enter those same totals on the total line.

Total number screened: Total number screened during the reporting period at each grade level.

Screened with glasses: Number screened with glasses on. (This number is a part of the total number screened.)

Number failed: Number who failed the screen or were referred for observable signs or symptoms. (This number should include those who fail other types of vision screens such as those used with stereoscopic instruments or other procedures, and at this time failure is determined by referral criteria associated with the particular screen.)

Failed not referred: Those who failed but are currently under an eye specialist's care *or* those who have an uncorrectable condition (enucleated eyeball, etc.).

Examined by eye specialist: After examination by an eye specialist the following breakdown of results should be reported:

No problem or treatment: Those referred who had no visual problem or who received no treatment for an existing condition.

Treatment or observation: Those referred who are receiving treatment from an eye specialist or whose conditions are being observed for a period of time.

Referred, no follow-up: Those referred who did not see an eye specialist or who were lost to the screening program. (This simply means that follow-up was not possible because either the person referred did not see an eye specialist or the information on the referral was unobtainable.)

REMEMBER: Calculate totals for each column at the bottom of the form and *check* those totals using the simple formula given, $C = D + E + F + G$. Also, note that columns E and F should be added together for a total examined by eye specialist.

Any questions about the proper use of this form can be directed to:

_____

_____

_____

STUDENT VISUAL ACUITY WORKSHEET

Name of pupil	Grade	Room	Screening instrument used — Snellen 10', Snellen 20', Ritmus, Keystone	Tumbling E, Stycar, Other	Results — Initial test	Date	Retest	Date	Referral date	Action

STUDENT VISUAL ACUITY WORKSHEET
(Filled-in sample)

Name of pupil	Grade	Room	Screening instrument used — Snellen 10', Snellen 20', Ritmus, Keystone / Tumbling E, Stycar, Other	Initial test	Date	Retest	Date	Referral date	Action
Johnny	3	14	Snellen 10'	pass	10/2				
Mary	3	"		fail	"		11/16	11/17	referred to Dr. Smith
Helen	3	"		quest.	"	fail	11/16	11/17	referred to County Clinic
Josh	K	2	Tumbling E						
Sue	K	2	"						
Betty	Sp. Ed		Stycar						
Tim	Sp. Ed		"						